Also by Jean Hegland:

The Life Within: Celebration of a Pregnancy

Into the Forest

Windfalls

STILL TIME

a novel by

JEAN HEGLAND

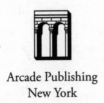

Arcade Publishing
New York

First Edition

This is a work of fiction. Names, places, characters, and incidents are either the products of the author's imagination or are used fictitiously.

Arcade Publishing books may be purchased in bulk at special discounts for sales promotion, corporate gifts, fund-raising, or educational purposes. Special editions can also be created to specifications. For details, contact the Special Sales Department, Arcade Publishing, 307 West 36th Street, 11th Floor, New York, NY 10018 or arcade@skyhorsepublishing.com.

Arcade Publishing® is a registered trademark of Skyhorse Publishing, Inc.®, a Delaware corporation.

Visit our website at www.arcadepub.com.
Visit the author's site at jean-hegland.com.

10 9 8 7 6 5 4 3 2

Library of Congress Cataloging-in-Publication Data

Hegland, Jean.
  Still time : a novel / Jean Hegland. — First edition.
     pages ; cm
  ISBN 978-1-62872-579-7 (hardcover : acid-free paper);
  ISBN 978-1-62872-617-6 (ebook)
1. Parent and adult child—Fiction. 2. Fathers and daughters—Fiction. 3. Dementia—Patients—Care—Fiction. 4. Domestic fiction. I. Title.
  PS3558.E419S75 2015
  813'.54—dc23   2015014025

Cover design by Georgia Morrissey
Cover photo: Trevillion

Printed in the United States of America

To the memories of
John Heminge and Henry Condell:
Reade him, therefore; and againe, and againe.

JOHN SENSES SALLY'S SADNESS as soon as he enters the room.

She is sitting on the sofa by the window, her head tipped to one side, her feet tucked under her as if she were a lass of sweet and twenty instead of a woman over sixty. But one glimpse of her hunched shoulders and the strained lines on her face tells him he cannot remember ever having seen her so forlorn.

Shocked by this vision of a grief so private John might swear he's had no inkling of it, he halts in the doorway, studying his wife. A sunset is gathering beyond the far green hills, a glorious mass of saffron, coral, and carnation clouds. Its rosy light burnishes her strong hands and silvered hair, but still she sits as if carved from marble, stricken and alone.

"Sweeting," John gasps, "my love." Gimping across the floor as fast as his bad hip will allow, he eases down beside her.

"What's the matter?" he asks, cupping her hand in his. By way of a gentle joke, he adds, "What villain hath done thee wrong?"

"Oh, John." She gives him a grateful smile. But then she sinks back inside her misery for so long that the sun is resting on the horizon before she whispers, "We have to talk."

She seems to be speaking more to herself—or perhaps to the

crimson sky—than to John, though he answers gallantly, "I trust we always will."

But instead of any of the discussion, debate, banter, or pillow talk that has served to make his time with her such delight, she launches into a bewildering thicket of reasons, facts, and explanations, a tangle so dense and prickly he finds he has to focus on her dear face and not her dire words.

Speaking too swiftly for him to follow, she outlines their expenses and their debts, mentions her business loans and pollination contracts, his pension and retirement accounts, the taxes on their house, their insurance premiums. But the terms and numbers whine so much like mosquitoes around his head that he has to resist the urge to swat at them.

From finances she skips to other things—stove burners left on, his tendency to wander, her sleepless nights—somehow binding all those disparate themes together and then investing them with a significance that eludes him no matter how he strains to attend.

"I wish we had more savings," she mourns, gazing dully at the ruddy clouds. "I wish I could retire. I wish we'd had longer together before this happened."

Her wishes stab him, leave him groping for a way to ease her pain. He gazes around the room, taking in the maple floors, the patterned carpets, the walls of books whose covers are more familiar to him than the veined and strangely wrinkled hand that strokes his wife's arm. Outside the window, at the bottom of the yard, he spies a row of Sally's hives, pale in the gloaming.

"If you have a bee in your hand," he offers, "what do you have in your eye?"

But Sally makes no effort to guess, and when he suggests, "Beauty," she answers with a smile so wan that it alone might stop his heart.

"Beauty is in the eye of the bee holder," he persists. "My beautiful bee holder," he marvels, gazing into her face. But instead of matching her smile to his, a stricken pain crosses her expression, and she closes her eyes for a moment as if summoning extra strength.

"What do you need?" he blurts. "What can I do?"

"Oh, John," she says again. Her voice is thick with gratitude, though the answer she offers him is enigmatical. She's found a place to help them, she claims, somewhere he will be safe while she is away at work, where he can stay so she will be able to get the sleep her doctor has told her she has to have.

Cupping his cragged face between her warm palms, she gazes directly into his eyes. "It's the last thing I want to do. I've tried and tried to find another way. I really don't believe we have a choice, but I want to make sure you agree." She looks at him imploringly, willing his answer to match her desperate need.

"For you," John replies, partly to forestall her further explanations, partly to soothe the worry in her face, but mainly because it is the simple truth, "I would do anything." He lifts her hand to his lips, bestows a kiss inside her calloused palm, then gently folds her fingers into a fist as if to keep his kiss cupped safe inside.

"It's a good place," she continues in a rush. "I'll visit every chance I get. I know they will take good care of you there." She pauses for a moment, as if seeking further strength. "Can you do this?" she pleads. "Are you sure it's okay?"

He is not certain exactly what she is asking of him, but it's clear what answer she needs to hear, and he gives it to her willingly, agreeing because he loves her, because he wants anything that troubles her to go away.

Borrowing words from *The Winter's Tale*, he tells her again what he told her at their wedding, "'I cannot be Mine own, nor any thing to any, if I be not thine.'" As the sun sinks to an incarnadine shard and ribbons of lavender fret the crimson clouds, he marvels yet again how perfectly the lines William Shakespeare wrote four centuries earlier for that young pup Prince Florizel fit what John is feeling now, as a man of seventy, half a world and four centuries distant from where that romance about severed families and second chances was first performed.

But Sally only sighs. Bending her head over their clasped hands, she whispers, "I'm afraid this will be so hard for you."

"I will be the pattern of all patience," he promises. Patting her hand, he vows, "I will endure."

Water wobbles in her eyes. With his finger, he daubs her tears. With his finger, he traces the path of a smile up her cheek, coaxes her mouth to follow.

For a long time they sit together inside the same silence, watching as the firmament glows with colors so strange and pure they seem to have been transported from another world.

"There's one more thing," Sally says when the final rim of sun has vanished behind the darkening hills, leaving a ruby ocean gleaming in its wake.

"Only one?" he quips.

"I'd like to get in touch with Miranda."

"Mir—?"

"Your daughter," she offers hastily, thus helping to forestall the vertiginous spin that has already begun in his chest and brain, that panic he feels more and more of late, when the simplest things—things he knows that he should know—seem to career beyond his grasp.

"Daughter," he echoes cautiously while half-formed images flicker in his mind—solemn toddler, howling infant, a child with a crayon in her hand.

Sally urges, "I really think Miranda needs to know what's happening."

"Miranda," John repeats, giving every syllable of the name that Shakespeare fashioned from the Latin word for "wonder" its due,

4

striving to subject even that single word to the kind of close scrutiny he has always taught his students is the best first step to studying any text. "Miranda."

"It could be good for both of you," Sally offers, "to be back in touch. I know you two've had your troubles. But London was ten years ago. A lot has changed since then. Miranda's a grown-up now, and you—" Catching herself mid-sentence, she reaches down to give John's knee a playful waggle. "You're getting old. Don't you think it's time to try again?"

A scowling teenager shoulders her way into John's mind, lavender hair bristling from her scalp as if she were an electrified porcupine. "I told you already," she snarls from the far side of the London taxi. "There's nothing more to say."

"I don't want to barge in where I don't belong," Sally continues while that hoyden glowers from her corner of the cab. "I've never met Miranda, and of course I can't promise anything, but I know you've missed her, and I really wonder if you two don't deserve another chance."

"Chance," John muses, offering the word like bait to the ocean inside his mind, waiting to see what it might net. The lines that come, though broken, are still luminous, yet another present from a lifetime of devoted study. *a chance which does redeem all sorrows* *comfort you with chance* *I, That have this golden chance and know not why*

But before he can identify which characters speak those words and in what plays, before he can think what those lines might possibly illuminate for him now, the sulking urchin has vanished from his ken, and in the sky the unworldly colors are fading, too, the rose muddying to rust, the delicate corals and lilacs graying into the inky welkin like thoughts dissolving.

"Is that okay, John?" Sally persists when it appears he is lost in those dimming clouds. "Would you mind if I tried to call Miranda?"

"I tried." He frowns. "I called her, but—"

"Can't you try again?"

He gropes in the shadows of his vanishing past, trying to find the plot or identify the motivations that might explain his current circumspection. "She cursed me," he announces in bitter wonder when the truth of it finally wafts into his awareness. "It's too late now," he tells the darkening world.

"Not yet." Sally grabs his hands and pulls them to her heart. "There's still time. You and Miranda could still forgive and—" She hesitates for a second, suddenly appears as abashed as if she had been about to say something untoward or even obscene.

"Forget," John offers when it seems she is unable to complete that simple cliché. "*Forget* is the word you're looking for, my love."

HE'S IN A ROOM. A plain clean room. A quiet clean cube of a room with a shining vinyl floor, pale green walls, still, odorless air. It's a room near monastic with its single bed, its simple dresser, two doors leading nowhere he would ever care to go. He is sitting in a strange clean room in the leather armchair he recognizes from his study at home—the same worn chair that has accompanied him through so many years and moves, so many other wives and former lives. He is sitting in his own familiar chair, looking out a wide window onto a green expanse of close-cropped grass bordered by an ivy-curtained wall.

It's a place he's never been—or seen, or dreamed—in all his life.

What country, friends, is this? That's what Viola asks, when, half-drowned by the storm that split her ship and doubtless killed her brother, she crawls from the surf onto some alien shore. Viola, John recalls, the sprightly heroine of Shakespeare's marvelous dark comedy *Twelfth Night.* Not Shakespeare's masterpiece, of course—since for the Elizabethans *masterpiece* would have meant the piece of work an apprentice used to gain admittance to his guild—but a magnum opus nonetheless, yet one more capstone for a career so wondrous it can only be called a miracle.

Outside, the sky above the wall that blocks his view is blue as eternity. It dizzies him to look on that much blue, just as it makes him dizzy to try to con where he is—so far from lecture hall, hotel room, or home—in what strange cell, walled in beneath what endless sky.

What country, friends, is this?

"It's a good place."

It was Sally who said that. Sally, his own dear wife, his last and best, sitting beside him on the sofa in their living room, her sweet face knotted with feelings it troubled him to see. Sally, holding his hand so tenderly in both of hers, her voice tight with worry as she explained and outlined and proposed. Sally, searching his eyes for the assent she needed to find there.

It was hard for him to follow her reasoning, hard even to identify the matter they were supposed to be discussing, but even so, he'd nodded solemnly, said, "Anything for you," assured her he would be the pattern of all patience, that he would endure.

But that was King Lear, roiling toward his madness. And he is John. John Wilson. John Hubbard Wilson, PhD, who has sworn to bear this strange shift in fortune for his own dear Sally's sake.

run through fire I will for thy sweet sake   *for your sake Am I this patient log-man*   *wish, for her sake more than for mine own, My fortunes were more able to relieve her*   The lines and phrases come to him like breaths, like gifts—sometimes popping full-blown into his mind, sometimes meandering through his thoughts like smoke from smoldering incense, curling into meanings that shift and morph, luring him on, drawing him in, tantalizing and compelling him as he sits in this unfamiliar room, watching, waiting, remembering. Still trying to understand.

"He who ends with the most understanding wins." At a certain point in his Introduction to Shakespeare classes, John always announces that. And then, standing in easy command at the helm of the lecture hall, holding his students in thrall with that mix of passion and iconoclasm he has perfected over half a century, he will go on to explain, "It's one of the most consistent lessons in all of Shakespeare's work. We see it in his comedies where his characters have to learn about themselves before they can earn their partners and their rightful places in society. We see it in his romances, where his characters come to comprehend the power of forgiveness and life's preciousness.

"And we see it even more clearly in his great tragedies. King Lear, Hamlet, Macbeth, Othello—there's no denying those guys live flawed lives and die unhappy deaths. But they do not die in their sleep. They do not die ignorant of either their own follies or of life's worth. Instead, they die in the fullest possible knowledge of who they are, of what they lived for, of the mistakes that they have made. As Shakespeare reminds us time after time, we're all gonna die. It's what happens while we live that's got to matter—what we learn, what we know, what we come to understand before we go."

Sometimes a memory envelops him. The clacketing of a typewriter. Rain pocking a dusty road. Another gust of laughter sweeping a lecture hall. Often those memories are shadowed things, wisps and ghosts that dissolve even as he tries to reach for them. But occasionally they arrive in his mind as precise as stories—memories polished by decades of remembering, their plots honed, their characters clear, their themes rich with meaning, remembrances so keen he sometimes feels he inhabits them more fully in retrospect than he ever did back when he was merely living them. He feels he can finally do those memories justice, now that he has lived longer and learned more, now that he has come to see how fickle it all is, how ephemeral, how much there is to be known and noticed and understood.

"I don't know where to go," a voice announces at his back. It is a woman's voice, rough with age. Like one of the abused queens in *King John* or *Richard III*, it hints at hidden sorrows. Despite the pang in his bad hip, John twists around in his chair to watch as the speaker shuffles into the room through the wide doorway that opens onto a bland bright hall.

"Is this where we are?" she demands. Her blouse sags from her jutting shoulders, her pant legs flap like sacks around her scrawny thighs.

"Begone," John growls. "Avaunt."

Ignoring him as if he were mere furniture, she circles the room until her attention is snagged by a pair of photographs that sit atop the dresser.

"What are these doing here? We don't even know these people," she complains, snatching up the nearest picture, and frowning at the image it contains. As if to prove her point, she holds the photo out toward John, tilting it to reveal a school portrait of a child—a girl of eight or ten—her pigtails askew, her gap-toothed grin at odds with the pinch of worry in her brown eyes. Like an old bruise or a dimming sunset, the photograph's colors have begun to fade, but even so, the sight of that grinning girl evokes in John a deep and complicated ache, provokes a yearning he can't quite locate or explain.

"Leave," he commands, his voice that can captivate a lecture hall full of freshmen swelling with authority. "Depart."

Shifting the photograph so she can gaze into the schoolgirl's eyes, the woman frets, "Why does everyone leave their messes for me? It's not firm, it's not defensible."

She sighs, "They brought me here to help me, my boys did." Disregarding John, she speaks to the photograph, the peevishness melting from her expression the longer she studies the girl captured there. "They said I just needed a little extra . . ."

Bewilderment fuddles her face. "Why am I here?" she asks the smiling paper girl. "I don't remember."

The photograph still dangling in her hand, she drifts out of the room. In the stillness she leaves behind, her final words seem to ripple outward like waves of water from a thrown stone—*don't remember don't remember don't remember don'trememberdon't*

"Remember?" Sally is always prompting him, "Don't you remember?" And although she asks it gently, he's nearly grown to resent her implication that remembering is a decision he might choose to make, that by forgetting he is being purposefully rash or slovenly.

Remember where you left your wallet. Remember where you put the car keys. Remember what the bank statement said. Remember what we did over the weekend, where we're going for dinner tonight. Remember to lock the door, to put away the ice cream, to turn off the stove. Remember that time in Sicily, and what we did in Rome, and where you left your jacket, your shoes, your address book. So many remembers, chattering like a rain of hailstones, bruising his head.

Remember your bold life   Remember since you ow'd no more to time
Than I do now   Briefly thyself remember
    pray you, love, remember

"Member to get me," he hears a child say. He sees her, too, floating somewhere in that odd darkness inside his head, a girl of five or six with crooked pigtails and a worried expression in her eyes. Gazing through the window at the walled greensward, John watches as she climbs out of the backseat of the car he has just pulled up to idle beside the curb.

"Member?" he quips, twisting around in the driver's seat. "Don't you mean *re*member?"

"No," she answers, lugging a pink backpack off the seat and shrugging into it. Shaking her head earnestly, she insists, "Member. *Re* means you have to do it again, like Mommy when she forgets. I want you to member the first time. I don't like to get forgot."

He feels a wisp of regret or even worry, but he knows he mustn't infect the girl with his concerns about her mother. "I'll *member* that!" he answers heartily.

Nodding solemnly, the child pushes the car door closed. Flooded by his love for her, John watches as she trudges across the schoolyard until she is lost among the other children. When he drives away toward campus and the classes and committees waiting for him there, he is certain he will never forget the promise he has just made, certain he'll not forget the quaint endearing charm of her request.

But stranded as he is in this strange chamber, that promise plagues him. He'd pledged to member that grave girl, but he has no idea where she might be waiting, no idea how to find her, or even exactly who she is.

Besides, he suddenly recalls, it was she who forgot, not he. He'd waited up all night for her—or at least for some sullen ghost or prickly older sister of that girl. For hours he'd stalked circles in the sitting room of their suite in the hotel off King's Road, breaking off his pacing to gaze out over London and wonder where in that whole huge city she might be, while the minutes ticked on toward morning and the hour of his speech.

She got lost. That's what she explained after the constables delivered her to the hotel the next evening. Speaking so defiantly it was as if it were he who had caused the trouble and not she, she insisted she'd just gone out for a little walk. She'd meant to be back before John and Freya returned from *As You Like It,* but she'd met some people in Trafalgar Square, some students. They'd gone to a pub, and maybe she'd had a bit too much to drink—she, who was still too young to drink in California. She got lost trying to find her way back to the hotel. She'd forgotten the hotel's name and what street it was on.

It was she who forgot, John reminds himself with a curt nod. It was her forgetting that cost them all so exceedingly.

Outside the window, the sun shines on. A row of flowers sways and nods at the base of the bushes that line the ivied wall. In the welkin above, a jet plane inches through the blue, leaving a wake of vapor as white and soft as the puffs of cotton his mother used to pull from the bottles of the pills she had to take. There was a window in that house, too, he remembers—in the house where he was born—a wide, modern window that his father had installed to underscore his standing as owner of the town's largest hardware store. A picture window is what his mother called it. In California's Central Valley, when telephones were affixed to walls and horses delivered milk.

The Johnny he was back then could stand at that picture window for hours, hands clasped behind his back, chin resting on the sill, his breath occasionally obscuring his vision with its warm fog while he gazed and gazed, soaking up the passing pageant one image at a time—a boy on roller skates, a car with fenders plump as pillows, a dog pausing to make water against the fire hydrant—the whole street his to study as long as he was good.

Though even then it was sometimes hard to know what that meant—*good*—hard to know how to be good right. And hard to know when what he had done was wrong. Sometimes his father growled and sometimes his mother squealed. Sometimes they purred. Inexplicably.

He'd had a dolly—he remembers—a puppy hand sewn and stuffed, given him by an aunt who ignored the injunction against letting boys have anything soft to love. Happy Dog. He'd named his dolly Happy Dog, and it was made of brown corduroy, with two black eyes embroidered on its long brown face. He slept with it at night, carted it with him during the day by one loose leg. Sometimes, watching out the window, he surreptitiously sucked a satin ear. Alone inside his own small body, gazing at the world.

Trying to understand.

In his intro classes, after he's said his piece about learning and knowing and understanding before we go, he likes to pause, to wait until his students have nodded their easy agreement and are bending back over their notebooks before he adds, "But it's really not that simple, is it? Because only the fools among us fail to realize how imperfect human understanding is. Anything we think we know about a situation or someone else or even ourselves is always limited by that old trap, point of view. Just as we are all of us stuck in time, so we are also stuck inside ourselves, doomed to live and die inside our own thick skulls.

"As Brutus says in *Julius Caesar*," he'll continue, borrowing the lines as effortlessly as if the words were his own, "'the eye sees not itself But by reflection.' And though here we might pause to admire how deftly Shakespeare makes the word 'reflection' earn its keep by suggesting both mirrors and contemplation, we also have to admit that what Brutus is saying is not really very profound."

Into the listening silence, he offers, "We can never see our own faces directly, never look straight into our own eyes. If it weren't for photographs, films, and mirrors, the only clues we would ever have about how we appear to other people would have to come from those people themselves."

In a good lecture, timing is everything, and here John has learned to pause while his students contemplate those thoughts—at first dismissing them and then resisting them, and then, when they recognize their truth and start to get an inkling of their import, nearly losing themselves in their vortex—before he suggests, "Only imagination allows us any relief from the trap of ourselves. Only imagination can give us any chance of seeing anyone else's self or soul.

"And it's art and literature—and Shakespeare—" he adds for the sake of the appreciative fond chuckle that ripples through the lecture hall, "that lets us imagine the humanity in other people, and helps us find it in ourselves."

They have so much to learn, his students. So much still to understand about ambiguity and interpretation and where meaning lies, so much to figure out about comedy, tragedy, history, and romance, too—both the tangled affections of their own sapling hearts, as well as those plays that critics call the romances, those radiant strange plays that William Shakespeare wrote at the end of his career.

It has grown harder, over time, to teach his students anything, what with so much else competing for their attention—new technologies along with ancient hormones—and the value of an education all but forgotten in the scuffle for a job. These days, even proper punctuation and correct citations are a challenge for some of his students. But John has never given up on teaching. Unlike many of his colleagues, he never lost his faith in students nor his passion for his subject. He never lost his conviction that studying William Shakespeare can help people live richer lives.

It's no longer a popular view. At least in academic circles the belief that human beings are capable of growth and change, and the faith that art can help to fuel those evolutions, have fallen far from favor. Nowadays, human beings are seen as little more than preprogrammed machines, or mere animals at the mercy of language. And humanism— that transcendent vision that spans centuries and religions in its celebration of reason, responsibility, art, and examined lives—has been tossed out like old bathwater, leaving humanity naked and shivering on the dirty ground.

He blames his colleagues for this disgrace—the younger ones for embracing it and the older ones for not resisting more. And he blames himself, too. He'd had his golden chance, that time in London. But fate confounded him, and all his efforts came to naught. People failed him, too, he reflects now with a scowl, letting him down in such troublous ways that he has long made it a practice not to think on them at all.

The room in which he sits is so silent he can hear time's tick, the small click of it rising from the watch that is strapped to the wrist resting in his lap. It's a wrist he can hardly accept as his, so startlingly sharp are its bones beneath such tissuey skin. The watch is more familiar—the good Elgin his father gave him when he graduated from high school. For over half a century it has counted out his seconds like a second pulse, though rarely has it been quiet enough for him to hear its beat.

Outside the window a tree keeps watch, its branches ticking in a whiff of breeze, its new leaves like crumpled petals unfurling. Mid-morning light filters through its limbs and leaves, casting a lace of shade across the ground outside, the floor within, his sneaker-shod feet. Studying those trembling shadows, John tries to discern patterns or tease out meanings, strains to find a way to understand this strange new story. But it is as if some essential piece were lost, a gap in the narrative, a lacuna in the text, the missing phrase or page he needs to make sense of the whole.

What country, friends

There was a clock in his fourth grade classroom, a little ticking one that sat like a round black gnome on the teacher's desk. He remembers watching it watch over time. Or rather, time doubles back so that he is there still—little Johnny Wilson, twisting and fidgeting in his seat as that clock taps his days away one *ticktock* at a time.

He is hungry for stories even then, already craving the other lives that stories let him live. Peter Rabbit, Tom Sawyer, Winnie-the-Pooh. Long John Silver with his bottle of rum. Every book he rescues from his school's neglected library takes him beyond himself, and each time he returns to being simply John, he finds himself enlarged.

He is enlarged, too, by words, by their meanings and their sounds, by the way they lull or trouble or thrill him, the spells they cast. *Soporific. Mortified. Heffalump. Ingenious.* Whenever his teacher asks the class to look up definitions in the dictionary, it takes him twice as long as any other child because his attention is diverted by every other word his eyes land on. *Adamantine. Adaptable. Addlepated. Adore.*

When he and the girl he has adored all year are sent outside to clean erasers, he keeps them busy longer than necessary, smashing the gray pads together with an industry that makes the girl giggle, banging until not one more white puff can be coaxed to billow away into the pollen-laden air. When he leans in to kiss her, he is as astonished by his own audacity as he is by the unexpected softness of her cheek.

Back in this strange cul-de-sac of time, John shakes his head in fond amazement at that kiss. No one kissed in his home, or even much in the movies that long ago. And yet inside that moment it had seemed the inevitable next thing, to kiss when he lacked matter to speak. And so he'd pressed his lips against the girl's cheek and held his mouth there, waiting. But before anything more could happen, she'd pulled away, looking solemn for an instant and then giggling and skipping off, leaving him to cart all the erasers back into the classroom by himself, his pants smeared with chalk, his ears as hot as if he had been leaning against the radiator.

Youth's a stuff will not endure. Though of course he hadn't understood that then. Back then old age had been as hard to believe in as love had been a breeze. Slapping the teacher's erasers, kissing that soft cheek, he'd been boy eternal. He'd not believed he would ever grow up, had not believed that he would one day shave or drive, one day leave home. Back then, death had been easier to believe in than old age. Even decades beyond that day, when his waist began to soften, and the first white hairs appeared like maggots in his thick brown locks, he had still not really understood that he—John Hubbard Wilson—could ever actually be old. Not aching and sagging, not steeped in the million indignities of a body gone soft and stiff, a brain gone, too. *Sans teeth, sans eyes, sans taste, sans every thing.*

"Good morning, John," a voice sings in his ear. "Remember me?" A woman plants herself in front of him, a hale woman, rotund and ruddy-cheeked as a country shepherdess—a Dorcas, a Mopsa, or a Phebe.

"Morning," she says again, reaching down to place a hand on his shoulder as if she were a pastor or a used car salesman. "I'm Matty. Yesterday I said I'd see you again tomorrow. And here it is tomorrow— and here I am!" A small gold cross hangs from a chain that is nearly lost in the folds of her plump neck. On the fabric of her tunic, green and pink kittens lick ice cream cones and nap on beach towels. The badge pinned to her tunic announces MATTY.

"How are you this fine day?" she asks when John does not respond. "How are you feeling?"

"When will I be leaving?" John asks briskly, ignoring her foolishness about feeling. "I've been waiting all morning."

"Oh, I'm not really sure," she replies with vague good cheer.

"I need to know," he insists. "I've got work to do. I've already waited patiently, more than . . . long enough."

"But you only just got here," she announces jovially, "yesterday."

"Yesterday?" he echoes, his voice wobbling on the word. He tries again, "What country is this?"

"What country?" Her laugh rings loud. "This is America, John. The good old USA. Solano, California. You moved across town, is all. It's just a little extra confusing right now because it's all so new. Moving's disorienting for anyone. Give it a little more time, and you'll get in the swing."

"I don't want the swing," he answers. "I want to leave. Where is my . . ." he pauses, searching for a worthy word, "Sally?"

"Your Sally?" The woman chuckles as if he'd intended another joke. "You mean, your wife?"

"Yes, yes, of course," he says impatiently, "wife." On his tongue that little syllable conjures a specific flavor of breath and flesh, evokes a certain frequency, a hum as warm and known as home. *Wife.* She'd been sad when he last saw her, her countenance seemed crushed, her spirit, too. It troubles him to recall. He worries that he is helpless to help her, imprisoned as he is in this confounding cell. Wherever she is, in whatever home or room or confine of her own, he hopes she is faring better now than he.

"She said this is an extra busy time of year for her, what with her bees and all." The blithesome woman gives a stout shudder. "But you

18

probably know that. She'll come to visit just as soon as she can. In the meantime, she's already called this morning to check on you."

"There's work I need—" John begins.

"Oh, forget about work, why don't you?" the woman interjects. "You've been working hard for years. You've earned a vacation. Why not just relax and enjoy a little break?"

"I've broken long enough," he snaps. "Please," he blurts, his voice startling even him with its raw pleading.

Something wavers in the woman's eyes, though she answers with practiced aplomb, "Let's give it a little longer before we start making any new plans. We'll take good care of you here—I promise. Your Sally will come to visit as soon as she can. And, hey—right now it's time for your meds."

"Meds?" John echoes, making the word sound silly.

"You know—medication. Medicine," the woman explains, holding out a little paper cup, shaking it so John can hear the rattle of the pill it contains.

"'No med'cine,'" he replies.

"Now John, you've got to take your medicine."

"'No med'cine in the world can do thee good,'" John continues, looking past his companion to the ivy-shrouded wall as he repeats Laertes's words to the dying Prince Hamlet.

"Sure it can," she answers reassuringly. "It's for your blood pressure."

When she leans down in front of him, John sees the concern hovering on her face, and for a moment he is tempted to sink into her solicitude, but then he waves it away with a wafture of his hand. "'In thee there is not half an hour's life,'" he continues, speaking Laertes's urgent eulogy for the sake of its own magnificence, speaking to himself since it is obvious this cheery rustic cannot understand.

"'The treacherous instrument is in thy hand,'" he adds, savoring the odd comfort of those stark words, imbued as they are with all the nuances of meaning and feeling they have collected throughout his decades of living with that play, so that now, like the layered colors of a Flemish painting, they seem to shine in his mind with their own internal light.

"It's a pill in my hand, John. I need you to take it." Her voice is as determinedly patient as if she were speaking to a child. "This isn't such a bad place," she says as she tips the little capsule into John's palm, watches while he places it on his tongue, and then offers him a glass of water. After he has swallowed and returned the glass to her, she reaches to take up his other hand, which has been lying loose in his lap like a possession he forgot he owned. "You'll like it here fine," she says, giving his fingers a little squeeze, "once you've gotten used to it."

But he stays silent, still basking in *Hamlet*, the pity and the horror and the stunning beauty of that play. After a moment, the woman returns his hand and moves away.

"Oh, hey—" she exclaims as she reaches the door, "I totally forgot! This'll cheer you up." Pausing in the threshold, she announces, "Your daughter called this morning."

John gives a little start. "My . . . ?" he echoes.

"Daughter," the woman fills in for him. "She wanted to know about visiting hours, and I told her there aren't any—visitors are welcome anytime. That'll be nice, won't it?—something to look forward to— seeing your daughter."

She gives the door frame a pair of quick taps as if she were firming the soil over a seed, and then she's gone, leaving John alone with a new set of words to rove his mind like changeable weather. *your daughter fair daughter pensive daughter daughter and heir daughter of most rare note a whoobub against his daughter where hast thou stow'd my daughter?*

"I think we've found your daughter." That's what the taller of the constables announced when John opened the door of the hotel room to find Miranda slumped between them, pale and stricken but glowering even then.

For a second his relief that she was alive trumped every other feeling. But after the constables left and he'd tried to get her to discuss where she'd gone and what she had done, she'd been much more stony than contrite, and even the next afternoon in the cab when he was returning her to Heathrow, she'd insisted there was nothing more to say. She'd apologized already, she claimed. She'd already said she'd never meant to be gone so long, had not wanted to make him worry or cause him any trouble. When he tried to help her see the inappropriateness of her actions and maybe even understand his side of the predicament and appreciate some of its awful consequences for him, she'd snarled and turned away.

He hated having to send her home, back to her increasingly ineffectual mother and another summer of small-time loitering with her semi-delinquent friends. But even if she hadn't chosen the night before his keynote speech to leave the hotel without asking, even if she hadn't kept him awake all night and worried for hours the next day, her misbehavior was much too grievous to overlook. From what little she'd revealed about where she'd gone and what she'd done, she was lucky that getting lost was all that happened to her. As both he and Freya had tried to impress upon her, things could have been much worse.

The three of them couldn't possibly have traveled on to Spain together after that—not with Freya so furious, and Miranda so sullen and unforthcoming, not with half a week of the conference still to go, and John desperate to curtail the ruin as much as possible. He knew Miranda hadn't had an easy time in the last few years, what with her mother getting more uncertain and her high school such a sham. But he also knew he wouldn't be doing his duty as her father if he failed to hold her accountable for her actions. Especially after her Tijuana escapade earlier that year, she needed to understand there were lines she wasn't allowed to cross. "Logical consequences" was what both Barb and Freya called it, and for once they were in agreement about the value of that approach.

"John," a voice trills from the hallway behind him. "It's time for arts and crafts. You want to join us? We're doing potato prints this morning."

But potatoes are an aphrodisiac, as every Elizabethan knows. And this morning John is not in the mood. "Pah," he says, batting at the air behind him with an impatient arm.

"You sure?" the voice wheedles. But he is too busy to trouble himself to answer. "Okay, then," the wheedler teases when he makes no further reply. "No art for you today."

But art doesn't mean potatoes. Art means knowledge or science or skill. Alchemy or entertainment. Magic. Trickery. Or transformation. Art can signify many things, but it is much too powerful for potatoes.

If this be magic, let it be an art Lawful as eating. It's Leontes who says that, John reflects, settling back into the lap of his chair with the satisfaction of a man who has just been served a plate of perfectly grilled steak. Leontes, the King of Sicilia, in the final scene of Shakespeare's great romance *The Winter's Tale*, as he and the daughter he has believed forever lost stand together before the marble sculpture of Hermione, Leontes's long-dead wife and the mother Perdita has never known, marveling at the stone's likeness to the woman she had been before Leontes destroyed everything.

It was Leontes who wrongly denounced Hermione as an adulteress, Leontes who ordered their newborn daughter Perdita abandoned as a bastard on the storm-chafed shores of fair Bohemia, Leontes who, in his misguided jealousy, tried to have his boyhood friend and Bohemia's king poisoned as his wife's seducer. Afterwards, it was Leontes's demented rage that caused the deaths of both Hermione and their dear son.

But during the sixteen years that have passed since then, Leontes has performed a saintlike sorrow, and in the previous scene, the audience has overheard how Perdita has been found, her royal birth revealed, her betrothal to Bohemia's Prince Florizel blessed, the kingdoms of their fathers united in friendship once again.

Now, precious winners all, they have assembled to view the statue of Hermione that the grave and good Paulina has kept hidden for so many years, and so excellent is the carver's art, and so great is Leontes's and Perdita's yearning, that when Paulina draws the curtain, both father and daughter must be restrained from kissing the freshly painted stone. A moment later, as they, their court, and the audience all watch in a hush of wonder, Paulina conjures music and commands the statue wake. And like unto an old tale or perhaps even a miracle, the sculpture quickens, the stone begins to breathe, and a living Hermione descends from her pedestal to embrace her husband, bless their daughter, take up her life again.   *Bequeath to death your numbness*   *Dear life redeems you   be stone no more*

It's been called the most moving moment in all of theater, the height of drama's art and Shakespeare's craft, the boldest and most beautiful scene he ever wrote. John has witnessed it many times onstage, has lived it many more times in the theater of his mind. He's wept, watching, more than once. He's even dared to call that scene sublime.

He tells his students that Shakespeare wrought one last miracle when he wrote his final plays—*The Winter's Tale, The Tempest,* and even *Cymbeline* and *Pericles*—those plays that Dowden dubbed romances for the way they begin with tempests, trials, and sundered families and end in scenes of recognition, with lives redeemed, worlds restored, and generations reunited.

Some critics have complained that Shakespeare's romances are too feeble or too fanciful to be taken seriously, that their gaudy plots, flimsy characters, and fabulous endings are evidence of an author grown careless, sentimental, or even senile. But John has long maintained that Shakespeare's final plays are not failures but new directions. Beyond *Hamlet*'s silence and *King Lear*'s howl and *Othello*'s suffocating darkness, beyond the intellectual intricacies and sour humor of the problem plays, William Shakespeare found one last transcendent vision. Beginning awkwardly in *Pericles* and *Cymbeline* and concluding masterfully in *The Winter's Tale* and *The Tempest*, he created yet another revolution, writing plays that celebrate the triumph of art and the gift of second chances.

Outside, the flowers begin to wobble, testament to a passing breeze. Tulips and daffodils, their shapes as simple as Easter eggs and shooting stars, their colors crayon bright against the green bushes that line the wall.

A child appears in John's mind's eye, a girl of seven or eight, sprawled on the floor of his office with a crayon in her hand. He keeps those crayons in his desk drawer for her visits, to occupy her while he works. "Draw me something," he'll suggest before turning his attention to whatever lecture or article or conference presentation he needs to finish next.

"What should I draw?" she asks, crayons scattered on the floor around her like a broken rainbow.

"Draw Romeo," he answers absently, or, "How about Falstaff?" or, "Try Lady Macbeth."

"What's a Falstaff?" or "Who's she?" she queries once or twice, but when she sees he is already too engrossed to answer, she invents answers of her own, hunched over her sheets of onion skin typing paper, as intent on her project as John is on his.

"Look," she commands when she is finished, and John will interrupt his work to admire the image she offers to his view—perhaps a pig with a curled tail, a wizard in an indigo cape, or a woman in a long magenta gown, each drawing labeled with spelling as eccentric as an Elizabethan playwright's: *ROMeO. Fol staf. LaDie MekbeT.*

Gazing at the dancing flowers, John feels a little shiver of pleasure, another flush of pride, remembers studying those endearing drawings and imagining how far that child would go.

But where? he asks the daffodils. Where did she go? It seems such a simple question. He can sense its answer shimmering just beyond his reach, and yet when he tries to grasp it, or to link those moments in his office with any part of now, his thoughts diffuse like smoke in wind, leaving only a faint bitterness behind, that awful nagging knowledge he's had too often of late that his failure to keep track of some fact or other is adding to all the disasters that still await him.

It will come to him again, he hastens to reassure himself. In an effort to prevent the panic that's already starting to strangle him, he promises himself that that girl's identity will resume its rightful place inside his mind as lost people and facts and places usually do, sometime when he is least expecting it—late at night, perhaps, or while he is driving down the freeway or in the shower, or even when he is trying to remember something else. He has known so many people in his life, has read so much and written so much, accomplished and experienced so much. It's understandable if he can't always remember every little thing.

It doesn't matter. That's what people tell each other when they forget. When a student raises her hand in class only to have forgotten what she wanted to say by the time it's her turn to talk, when a colleague stops John in the hall to tell him he read an article he thought John might be interested in though he can't at that moment recall the author's name, when Sally says there was something she wanted to ask him but now she can't remember what, they laugh and shrug and reassure each other, "It doesn't matter, it wasn't really important—or if it was important, it will come back later."

It will come back later—John muses out the window—embodying the romantic view of time, the belief that the future will restore what's lost, that nothing that truly matters is ever gone for good.

"John," a woman says, breezing in, "Are you ready to go—?"

"Certainly," he answers with alacrity, planting his palms on the arms of his chair and preparing to stand.

"—to lunch?"

"I've no need to eat," he replies as he levers himself upright. "I'm ready to go right now."

"To lunch," the woman agrees, reaching out a hand to steady him. She is a well-cushioned lass somewhere on the far side of thirty. Her top is decorated with images of frolicking kittens, and the tag on her chest reads MATTY.

"Not lunch. I've been waiting all—" He breaks off, suddenly lost in a swirl of confusion in which the facts of his situation—how long he has been waiting, and for what or whom—spin past just out of reach. "A long time," he adds more feebly.

"I'm sorry about that," the woman replies. "But hey—your wait's over, 'cause now it's time to eat."

"There's been a mistake. I need to speak with . . . whomever is in charge. I don't belong here. I understand it's not your fault," he offers generously. "But we need to resolve this before the situation grows worse."

"Okay," she agrees. "How about you eat first, and then we'll see?"

"See what?" John shoots back. Pleased by his sudden acumen, he adds, "What will we see?"

"First of all, we'll see what's on the menu. Whatever it is, it's sure been smelling good."

This is chopp'd logic, John knows. He resents the evasion of it, the equivocation. But he suddenly feels too dizzy, too confused and ill at reckoning to challenge it. Instead he suffers the woman to lead him down a long bright hall to where a ragtag group of diners is converging by the French doors at the far end, some with walkers, some with canes, several riding in wheelchairs, some arriving like shy guests, some smiling vaguely like expectant hosts who've forgotten exactly whom they invited to dinner, others sour-faced or with faces absent of expression, all of them shuffling into a dining room where kitchen aides are filling water glasses and placing baskets of rolls around.

His attendant shows John to a table set for four. "How's this?" she asks, pulling out a chair, steadying him as he plops down. Two grandams already sit in the chairs on either side of him. The stout one waits placidly, hands folded in her lap, her head bobbing as if she were keeping time to a secret music. Opposite her, a bone-thin woman bends over to study the framed photograph in her lap.

"That's Esther," John's escort announces, gesturing toward the portly dowager, "and this is Betty," she adds, reaching down to stroke the gaunt one's arm. "Ladies, you don't mind if John joins you two?"

The skeletal woman does not respond, but the other interrupts her nodding to shake her head no, making a complicated motion with her head like a mobius strip. "Tea for two," she sings, "and two for tea." Raising her hand from her lap, she swings it like a conductor's baton, keeping time to her shred of song.

"John is new here," Matty explains.

"How do you do?" John says, urbane and wary.

"How do I do what?" the quiet woman whispers, her head bent over her lap as if she were asking the photograph.

"And here comes Robert," Matty announces as if it's welcome news. Turning to the hound-faced man who is easing himself down into the chair across from John, she asks, "How are you today, Robert?"

"Okay, okay," he replies mournfully. "Whatever you say, dear. Did you bring my shovel?"

Elsewhere, other residents are settling in at other tables. Small arguments flare up about who will sit where, with whom. One man calls another man a bastard, says he's been out to get him from the start. A woman sitting nearby chuckles merrily, announcing to the room at large, "I keep thinking there's something I need to be doing wrong."

At a corner table a tiny crone in a white blouse and full dark skirt sits weeping. Occasionally she moans a few words in a language that John does not recognize—something Eastern European, perhaps—not Russian, but an even throatier cousin. But no one speaks to her, and soon her weeping becomes another background sound, like the clatter from the kitchen, like Frank Sinatra's crooning about how fairy tales can come true that leaks from the speakers in the corner of the room.

An aide moves among the tables with a bottle of hand sanitizer, squirting a dollop onto each diner's palm. There is a little flurry of busyness while they rub the goo between their fingers. An antiseptic floral smell fills the room.

"A termite walks into a bar," the man across from John announces, "and asks, 'Is the bar tender here?'" The man looks like an aged tortoise, his gaze fixed, his lashless lids hardly blinking. "An apple pie walks into a bar," he continues in a solemn monotone, "and the bartender says, 'Sorry, we don't serve dessert.'"

While his guests were finishing their dessert at his retirement dinner, John unwrapped the gifts they'd given him—a bobble-headed Shakespeare doll, a coffee mug emblazoned with curses from the plays, the framed cartoon an artistic graduate student had drawn of John genuflecting before the Roubiliac sculpture. Then he'd delivered quite a nice little speech, beginning by addressing his colleagues as *we few, we happy few, we band of scholars*, and going on to observe that although *emeritus* sounded like a disease, he hoped it wasn't fatal because, unlike Prospero, he wasn't nearly ready to drown his book.

Sitting down, he'd been bathed in genuine applause—and even a few huzzahs—and he'd gone home so warmed by his colleagues' show of esteem that he found himself rethinking several long-standing feuds. But before he could dive into his work, he'd had to play general contractor for the home renovation they'd been

28

planning ever since Sally moved in. Then his hip flared up again, and the doctors warned he shouldn't wait any longer to have it replaced, and once he finally recovered from the operation and completed the rehab, he'd been retired for over two years, and it was time for their trip to Sicily.

Sally wanted to meet Hyblean beekeepers and watch them work with their black Sicilian bees. She'd wanted to learn about beekeeping in mud hives and maybe help to harvest the honey that had been considered the world's finest for at least three thousand years, the honey that Shakespeare celebrated in his plays.

John hoped to develop his thinking about the evolution of drama by visiting the Greek theaters that dot Sicily's coasts and attending some authentic Sicilian puppet shows. With Sally at his side, he'd looked forward to strolling the streets in Siracusa where Plato and Sappho and Aeschylus had visited, the streets where Archimedes had rushed wet and naked from his inspired bath. He'd wanted to breathe and taste and view that mythical land that, like Denmark, Verona, Venice, and Bohemia, William Shakespeare had dreamed but never seen, the island where Benedick and Beatrice sparred and loved, where Leontes raged, and where his saintly wife Hermione bequeathed to death her numbness and was stone no more.

But instead of being stimulating, their trip seemed pointlessly complicated from the start. Even before they left home, planning and packing were more confusing than they had ever been before. He and Sally missed their connecting flight in Frankfurt for some frustrating reason John never entirely understood, and that first night, when they finally reached the hotel Sally had booked for them in Palermo, John opened his suitcase to find it contained only underwear and socks. He'd had to borrow Sally's toothbrush, had had to find a business district the next morning and go shopping, joking with Sally until he nearly believed it himself that it had been his plan all along to buy a new wardrobe of Italian clothes.

It made John's head spin to be surrounded by people laughing and arguing in a language he could not understand. It wearied and irritated him, as if he were trying to live in a place of constant wind or blowing sand, and he'd even begun to suspect that Shakespeare's Italian prejudices were founded on something more substantial than hearsay and chauvinism. Sally turned as solicitous as the parent of a preschooler after he misplaced his wallet for the third time. But he'd found himself more irked than soothed by the patience honeying her voice, and her little quips about absentminded professors only caused him to become obsessed with keeping track of his possessions, so that he spent the rest of the trip patting his pocket every few minutes to check for his wallet, fingering his passport, clutching his camera strap even as they ate.

Even Sally's facility with Italian came to seem more like a wedge between them than a bridge, one more thing that placed her squarely in a world that had suddenly and inexplicably turned against him. In the end, he returned to California not invigorated but exhausted, to a house he barely recognized, the freshly painted rooms so unfamiliar that he got lost his first night home, trying to find the bathroom in the dark.

It was as if the plane they'd flown back to California on had somehow got diverted and returned them to an altered world, a place so similar to the one that was his native home that he could work his thoughts into a twist of knots trying to discern the differences, but another place nonetheless, a mazy place where nothing could be entirely trusted or assumed.

After Sicily, it seemed he could not quite get his life back into focus. Following a case of jet lag as debilitating as a month-long bout of flu, he'd at last turned his attention to setting up his office in the spare bedroom and been dismayed to find that the graduate assistant who'd helped him pack up his belongings at the university had fit the books and journals into boxes according to their size instead of preserving their order on his bookshelves.

But rather than let annoyance untemper him, he'd gone straight to work, patiently emptying all the boxes and stacking their contents in piles on the floor, tossing out the incomprehensible stuff that that idiot kid had mistakenly assumed he'd want to keep—old newspapers, programs for conferences decades past, even a strange sheaf of children's drawings with such confounding titles as "CaLLe BaN," "ROZlin," and "ROMeO."

He'd meant to start by arranging all the volumes whose authors began with *A* on the shelf next to his desk. But he soon became as confused as a freshman about editors and coauthors, and he began to wonder if maybe he shouldn't separate his books by play or century or subject instead. Finally, he decided to postpone organizing anything until he'd had a chance to get some writing done. Later, he promised himself, once he'd made some headway with his real work, he could return to the menial chores of housekeeping.

But writing, too, proved unexpectedly frustrating. He wanted to develop his arguments for the reclamation of humanism. But time and again he would begin with a promising hunch for how best to frame his thoughts only to find that when he tried to follow his thinking any further, his ideas seemed to either dissolve or grow infinitely more complicated, bifurcating until they had somehow connected with every other idea he'd ever had, interweaving with so many questions, musings, and epiphanies that he was left thrilled and bewildered in equal parts.

Several times he ran across drafts of other articles that addressed nearly the same material, but when he attempted to incorporate the two sets of thoughts, he discovered they left large gaps in his reasoning or offered subtle contradictions of each other, and any attempt to reconcile or reconnect them sent him back to the plays, back to other scholars, back to his leaning stacks of journals, his tumbling piles of books.

And all the while the mail kept coming, bringing more things that needed reading, needed sorting, required congratulation or rebuttal. Newsletters and journals continued to appear. Letters arrived from former students, asking for recommendations, sending monographs, or wedding, birth, or book announcements. But the names on the envelopes were meaningless, the faces in the photographs morphed into a single nameless face, and he set the letters and pictures aside until he had more energy to respond to them.

Until his mind could clear.

"An amnesiac walks into a bar," the rustic sitting opposite John gleeks, "and asks, 'Do I come here often?'"

"A pair of jumper cables walks into a bar, and the bartender says, 'I'll serve you as long as you don't start anything.'"

The plates the aides deal out around the table contain salads topped with slices of grilled chicken. John studies his food as if it were some sort of test or trap, the strips of pale meat, the dollops of dressing, the stiff romaine. Wisps of warning circle in his head—Tamora sitting down to the pie that she herself hath bred at Titus Andronicus's banquet table, the traitors in *The Tempest* preparing to partake of Ariel's bewitched feast, the gory ghost of Banquo claiming his place in Macbeth's dining hall—all the dangers of eating where one does not belong. He misses Sally's presence across the table, wonders if she's bothering with food at all, now that he's no longer there to keep her company. When he first met her, she'd been living on little more than bagels and smoothies, too occupied with trying to establish her apiaries and reclaim her life after her caddish husband's loutish departure to pause even long enough for a real meal.

"The food is good here," announces his plump table companion.

Reaching for her glass of milk, she adds cheerily, "No dessert until you drink your milk."

Warily, John takes up his own glass. He hasn't drunk a glass of milk since before his mother died. Now he takes a sip, lets its cold viscosity fill his mouth as his gaze travels the room, glancing from the busy aides to the other diners, their white or gray or bald heads bent over their food. Swallowing, he sets his glass back down, touches his napkin to his lips. The milk is not as foul as he had feared, and yet he wishes it were wine instead—a sprightly pinot blanc or a spicy zinfandel. Or perhaps the *vino nero* he and Sally discovered in Sicily—black wine to match Homer's wine-dark sea—and which they'd first tasted on the terrace of a restaurant overlooking the very waters where Odysseus wandered for so long.

"Do you want your chicken?" the stout woman asks, eyeing the strips of meat atop John's salad with a look akin to lust.

"Children?" the quiet one murmurs, still studying the photo in her lap.

For a long time he'd assumed their trip to Sicily would mark the boundary between the disappointing final chapter of his academic career and the commencement of the real work of his retirement. How much he would accomplish, he'd marveled in advance—how much he would read and write and publish, how much discover and create—in those open, golden days when his time would be his own and he would have no one to answer to but William Shakespeare, Sally, and himself.

Even after over half a century, each time he returned to any of the plays, he still noticed something new. Each line was an inexhaustible garden, every word its own rich trove, each plot so momentous and meaning-laden he knew he could never possibly be finished with it. In his retirement, he could finally work for himself—and for the work itself. He would publish in earnest, he promised Sally, before he perished for real.

How happy he would be in those calm, wide days. With Sally at his side—his fine and final wife. His last and best. After his disastrous marriage to Freya ended, he'd assumed that all he'd finally learned about how to husband would be for naught, since he would never have another chance of wiving at three score and some. But he'd found all the graces he'd ever desired in one woman at last, discovered her on a shining afternoon in early summer, balanced on a ladder propped against the maple tree outside his office window, while she coaxed a shimmering orb of honeybees from the branch where it dangled two stories above the ground.

She was wearing a veil that made her look like a cross between a Victorian dowager and an extraterrestrial alien, but when he opened his window the better to watch her ease the seething mass into the box that sat atop her ladder, he'd been amazed to see that her hands were bare. A moment later, above the hum and sizzle of all those thousands of bees, he'd heard a scrap of tune, and he'd realized to his astonishment that she was singing.

He was waiting at the bottom of her ladder when she descended, the box murmuring in her arms like a sleeping dragon or a captured melody. She was used to people stopping to watch when she caught a swarm, and her greeting was brisk but not unpleasant as she unzipped herself from her bee suit, pushed back her veil and shook out her silvered hair. Given her slender figure and her dexterity on the ladder, she was much older than John had expected, but he found himself pleased by that surprise. The friendly fans of wrinkles at the corners of her eyes and the veins on her strong, deft, naked hands made her somehow seem more fully human than the golden clones that filled his classes and his seminars. Even so, he'd felt as tongue-tied as Orlando upon first meeting Rosalind as he stood beneath the maple and stammered out some sodden-witted question about the dangerousness of bees.

"Dangerous!" she'd scoffed. "Don't you read the news? It's bees who're in danger, not me. Besides, a swarm of bees is about as docile as a cow. Easier to get out of a tree, too," she'd quipped as she carried the box toward her pickup and John trotted along beside her, already half-captured himself.

"Where is everyone?" she'd asked, when he appeared incapable of either departing or having anything sensible to say. "The campus looks deserted." She chuckled. "Usually I draw a larger crowd."

"We're between terms," he explained as she leaned over the wall of the truck bed to set the muttering box carefully behind the cab. "Spring semester's over, and summer session doesn't start until next week. I'm just here working on an article."

"An article?" She paused to give the box a brief caress. "About what?"

"Oh," he'd shrugged. "Just some thoughts about one of Shakespeare's plays."

"*William* Shakespeare?" she asked, as if there might be others. "Which play?"

"*A Midsummer Night's Dream*," he answered warily, already anticipating the inevitable awkward end to their conversation.

"I saw that just a few months ago!" she exclaimed. "They'd made the fairies gay," she added with a laugh. "The friends I went with had conniptions, but I liked it. In a funny way I thought it kind of fit.

"Let me ask you this—" she'd gone on more seriously. "The other day I read an article that said he was an impostor."

"Who?" John quipped, dreading what was coming next. "Bottom? Puck? Oberon?"

"No." She frowned. "Shakespeare. They said that someone else wrote all his plays."

It was a question he hated, the question he'd grown used to having to field far too often from the kind of tiresome student who also wanted to claim that the world had been created in six days and that global warming was a hoax. It was another reason he avoided revealing his profession to strangers on long-distance flights. But this woman did not strike him as a collector of conspiracy theories or an idiot or a snob, and so, as she swung her ladder from the tree, carted it across the lawn, and stowed it in the bed of her truck, he'd explained a few of the most glaring flaws in that boiled-brained claim that some other playwright, or some nobleman, or even Queen Elizabeth herself must have written—in his or her spare time, and without anyone suspecting it for the next two hundred and fifty years—the plays attributed to William Shakespeare.

"I thought that sounded like a loony theory," she said when he finished his polite polemic. "I'm glad it isn't true."

She smiled as if an interesting new thought had just occurred to her. "I don't know why it matters really. I mean, those plays are still those plays—aren't they?—whoever wrote them. But somehow it bothered me to think it was all some kind of hoax."

His heart already humming like a swarm of bees, John assured her that it was always good to see Shakespeare being taken seriously— even as his own impostor. Generously, he added that, misguided as the people were who claimed that no undereducated glover's son from some backwater village could have ever written *Hamlet* or *As You Like It* or *Othello*, they were only trying to make a miracle comprehensible. Especially in these anti-intellectual times, it was gratifying to see the value of a good education being championed so ardently. But what those naysayers failed to understand, John said, smiling into Sally's lovely, forthright face, was that no true miracle could ever be explained.

That smile is still illuminating his expression when someone jostles his shoulder and John looks up to find himself in the oddest banquet hall. When he glances down again, a bowl of ice cream has materialized on the table in front of him, a spoon tucked at a jaunty angle between the scoops.

"Oh, goody," the ancient matron beside him exclaims when a

similar bowl appears in front of her. "I'll get fat," she gloats, snatching up her spoon.

"'We fat all creatures else to fat us,'" John offers experimentally, "'and we fat ourselves for maggots.'"

"For maggots?" she asks, bewilderment crossing her face like a brief fog.

"Magic," corrects the fool sitting opposite him.

"Hamlet," John answers curtly, his hopes dashed. "When he refers to Polonius at supper—not where he eats, but where he is eaten. By a certain convocation of politic worms."

On their first date, he'd taken Sally to a production of *Hamlet* down in the city. "I've never seen *Hamlet*," she announced as he drove south through the sleek green hills. "In fact, practically the only thing I know about it is 'To be or not to be.'"

"That's not a bad place to begin," John replied mildly, suddenly dismayed at the thought of becoming even moderately smitten by a woman who knew nothing about *Hamlet*. Especially at his age, when the heyday in his blood was at least a little tamed, he'd assumed it would be good to have plenty of ready topics of conversation.

"So," Sally prompted after they'd driven a moment in silence, "I could use a rundown on how the story goes. I'm afraid I haven't yet had a chance to buy the CliffsNotes, professor."

He cringed almost as much at "professor" as he did at CliffsNotes, but when he glanced in her direction, he saw her expression was more playful than ironic, and so he'd responded in kind, by clearing his throat theatrically and straightening an imaginary tie. "When the play begins," he said, allowing his voice to settle into its professorial register, "Hamlet's father, the King of Denmark, has just died, and his mother has already married her dead husband's brother. If Hamlet weren't upset enough by this, a ghost appears claiming to be the spirit of Hamlet's dead father, and maintaining that he was murdered by his brother—"

"—who is now the king and married to Hamlet's mom—"

"—exactly, and saying that if Hamlet ever loved his father, he will revenge his death by killing his uncle, the new king."

"Sounds like we're off to a juicy start," she observed, craning her neck to study the winery they were passing, with its vast parking lot, drawbridge, and crenellated towers.

He smiled. "The rest of the play is about Hamlet trying to decide whether the ghost was truly the spirit of his dead father, and—if it was—whether revenge is really the right way for him to remember his father, and—if revenge is the right way—then how he should go about getting it. In the end—"

"—no spoilers, please!" She reached across the seat to give his elbow an impish tap. "I'm sure they all die, but I'd like to wait and see for myself how it happens."

Her hand lingered for a moment on his arm, and suddenly he found it oddly invigorating to be going to see *Hamlet* with someone who did not know how the play ended, especially when she added, "What I'd really like to know is what you think I should be paying attention to during the show."

It was a generous question, and as they curved through rolling vineyards where the summer's fresh vines twined across their rows like creatures caught in mid-dance, he savored the moment he took to choose a direction for his thoughts.

"Beginnings are important," he began, casting a shy look in her direction and then nearly blushing when his glance intersected with her direct gaze, "and, uh, also in literature, too, as auguries," he fumbled, "or suggestions of themes, intimations of what might be to come. In *Hamlet*, the beginning is so straightforward that many people hardly notice it. At first it might just seem like filler, simply a way to get the story going. But it's brilliant, really. Like practically everything else in that play, it's an invitation to—"

"Don't keep me in suspense," she said with a laugh, "how does it begin?"

"It begins with a question, and since the entire play is riddled with questions—unanswerable questions, most of them, enigmas that deepen the more one considers them instead of resolving—"

"But what's the question?" she insisted.

"'Who's there?'"

"'Who's there?' That's the beginning of *Hamlet*?" She chuckled. "Sounds like the middle of a knock-knock joke."

Grinning at the road ahead, John admitted, "I never thought of that."

She fell silent for a quarter of a mile or so, seemingly concentrating on some inward puzzle. Then, suddenly brightening, she exclaimed, "Toby!"

"What?"

"Toby—get it? 'Who's there?' 'Toby.' 'Toby who?' 'Toby or not Toby?'

"But why," she continued before he'd finished his appreciative groan, "do you say 'Who's there?' is a good beginning for the play?"

"Because it's a play about identity and appearances, about whether the ghost is a true messenger from Hamlet's father or a goblin damn'd from hell, and whether Hamlet is crazy or only pretending, and whether he loved Ophelia more than forty thousand brothers or whether he loved her not. It's a play about the difference between 'seems' and 'is,' and 'Who's there?' suggests all that. In the end—"

"Stop, stop!" She commanded, pummeling his jacket merrily. "Save the end for last. If nothing else, it'll give us something to talk about on the way home."

Someone is weeping. Behind him, in a corner of the hall, somebody has been crying the whole time he has been dining. Those cries rise and fall in his awareness like a distant alarm. It's a wearisome, worrying noise, both nagging and disturbing, and he thinks that someone should put a stop to it.

At his own table, his dining companions are finishing their ice creams, the jocund one cleaning her bowl as if she were completing some crucial quest. His own ice cream has softened into a gooey puddle while he's been away.

The weekend after *Hamlet*, Sally invited him to come with her while she visited one of her apiaries, which turned out to be simply a row of a dozen white hives set between a vineyard and a small green creek.

She'd brought an extra veil for him to wear and he stood beside her, watching through the mesh of it as she lifted the lid from the first hive box and pried off the inner cover. A cloud of bees came gusting up. He took an inadvertent step backwards, startled by both their numbers and their vigor.

"They're only saying hi," she said with a laugh as he edged further away, suddenly newly wary of the entire enterprise.

Standing over the open hive, Sally closed her eyes and inhaled deeply. "I love the smell of a happy hive," she said as she let out her breath.

"Can you smell it, too?" she asked, opening her eyes and turning to him, and when he moved a little closer, he was suddenly aware of the scent wafting from the hive—a clean rich smell like a field of ripe wheat, or an orchard at midnight, or the healthy smell of sex.

"Aren't they lovely?" she urged as he drew nearer. Prying inside the box with a tool like a miniature crowbar, she eased out a frame sizzling with bees. Holding it up for his inspection, she pointed out the honey, pollen, and brood hidden beneath the undulating mass of insects.

"It is a little intimidating," he admitted, glancing askance from that seethe of bees to her serene face.

She smiled at him beneath her veil. "I used to feel that way, too.

But now I find it calming. Bees'll tell you when you're not welcome. You just need to listen."

"What are they saying now?"

She paused for a moment, cocking her veiled head to one side as if to listen more intently. "They're just gossiping. They love to gossip."

"What are they gossiping about?"

She listened further. "You."

"And?"

"So far they say they like you fine."

While he tagged along beside her, she worked on down the row, opening hives, checking on brood patterns and honey stores, rearranging frames, stacking extra boxes on some of the hives, making other arcane adjustments for reasons she explained but that left him bewildered nonetheless. From several of the larger hives she decided it would be okay to take a frame or two of honey even that early in the season. Holding the frames she'd chosen above the open hives, she gave each one a short, sharp shake that dislodged hundreds of startled bees into the general buzz and whirl.

She pointed out forager bees returning to their hives, the bags on their back legs bulging with pollen. She showed him where on the frames they had already packed the comb with orange, red, or yellow pollen, and then she smiled happily when he observed that the glowing hexagons put him in mind of tiny stained glass windows. She showed him brood in different stages, from eggs like grains of sand to fat white larvae, and together they watched as a new bee struggled to break free of the cell in which her metamorphosis had occurred so she could join the life of her hive.

Sally said bees had to visit five hundred thousand blossoms to make a cup of honey, said that one bee would work her whole lifetime to produce less than a tenth of a teaspoonful of the stuff. Since no bee can survive more than a day without its hive, she explained it was really the hive that should be thought of as a single creature, and she told him it was possible for a healthy hive to live for centuries, replacing workers and drones and queens indefinitely. She mourned the current fate of bees, said some nights she could hardly sleep for worrying about their future.

"I never realized how much there was to beekeeping," he admitted as she was opening the final hive.

She gave him a keen glance from beneath her veil. "Kind of like *Hamlet*," she offered, lifting a frame from the top box and flipping it deftly to inspect both sides.

"I like to think of myself as more of a bee helper than a beekeeper," she added as she replaced that frame and drew out another, "since the bees generally keep themselves just fine. My job is just to help them along a little, make sure they have everything they need to thrive."

"And then *help* yourself to their honey," he teased.

"Actually," she answered stoutly, "if I'm doing it right, I'm really doing them a favor by carting off their surplus stores. Little misers," she explained affectionately, "they'll save up more honey than they need, and then waste energy trying to keep it warm and dry all winter.

"Though you have to be careful," she warned so ardently it was as if she expected he would soon be helping bees himself. "It's easy to kill a hive if you take too much honey. There's more art than science to it," she added with a small wry sigh, "and, like anything else that really matters, sooner or later it's bound to break your heart."

She'd packed a loaf of seedy bread, a blue-veined cheese, a basket of perfect apricots. He contributed a creamy chardonnay. Her work completed, they doffed their veils, spread a quilt beneath the twisting branches of a massive oak, sat munching and sipping, gazing down the tidy rows of trellised grapes while the bees droned and the stream gurgled and the sun dappled down through the leaves and lichened branches.

Sitting in that drowsy yard, he felt saturated by his awareness of the woman beside him, her quiet breath, her worn hands, her amiable wrinkled face. He felt attuned and charmed, drawn to her in a dozen different ways, but also utterly foolish. He was sixty-four. He had not touched a woman in the nearly three years since Freya left, and for all that time it had seemed absurd to think he would ever touch a woman again.

Casting surreptitious glances in Sally's direction, he felt more awkward than he ever had before in the presence of a woman he fancied, as if all his previous experience had taught him nothing about courting except how fraught it was. He was so much more aware of his own inadequacies, too, of how old and raw and doltish he really was. As he helped himself to another apricot, he determined it would be wiser to enjoy this woman's friendship than hazard all for any other prize.

"Ready for dessert?" Sally asked when their glasses were empty and the cheese was gone. And almost before he could nod, she had hopped up and was returning with a frame of honey, a few bees still clinging to its fat gold cells. Like a girl wiping a fingerful of cake batter from a bowl, she pressed her forefinger down into the comb, smashing the waxen seals so that honey oozed up.

"Another thing people don't realize about honey is that there's a tremendous variety of color and flavor. It's like wine," she said, glancing at the field in front of them, "but even more so. Every frame captures a particular season and location, what flowers were blooming when."

Lifting her dripping finger toward his mouth, she commanded, "Taste."

Her gesture was as direct and matter-of-fact as the scent of her work-warmed body, but still it caught him off guard. He felt absurd but also oddly virginal as he closed his mouth around her honeyed finger and sucked its sweetness, trying to tease out every particular flavor she was offering him.

"Yum," he hummed, smiling into her face as he opened his lips to release her finger.

"Dig in," she suggested with a happy grin, swiping her finger back along the groove of broken, oozing comb, and signaling him to do the same.

After they'd had their fill of honey still warm from the hive, she'd lifted her finger to her own mouth one final time.

"Watch this," she commanded as she daubed her lips with honey.

"Watch what?" he asked after a bemused moment in which he'd admired the bones of her cheeks and her deep-set eyes.

"You have to wait," she admonished, smiling as serenely as a living version of the ancient kore sculptures they would later admire in Sicily together. "Be patient."

They waited for a long time then, he slightly puzzled and she utterly serene, while the bees danced around the hives like living bits of light, and the oak's new leaves danced in the dallying breeze, and scraps of lines wove their own dance in his head—*Where the bee sucks, there suck I,* and, *Merrily, merrily shall I live now,* and, *Not like a corpse . . . But quick and in mine arms.*

When a bee landed on Sally's lips, he gave an inadvertent gasp and reached over instinctively to brush the insect away. But she touched his hand to stay his gesture. Her smile never changing, he'd watched, disconcerted and enthralled, as the bee traversed her lips, its cellophane wings folded across its back while its legs and antennae wobbled busily and its proboscis probed her smile, reclaiming the sweetness it had discovered there. Sally's eyes met his. She hugged his hand with hers, and her smile grew as the bee continued its progress unhampered.

When the bee finally flew off, she laughed merrily. "It tickles," she announced, licking her lips, and then rubbing at the tickle with her hand.

"That takes courage," he answered, bemused but also entranced.

"Maybe," she replied. "And maybe it's worth it," she added, moving her bee-kissed mouth toward his.

"This is a nice party," a stout dame announces, yanking John from that golden moment to deposit him in some wrong present where he sits with a motley assortment of messmates in a dismal dining hall. "But I think we should go to my place next," the woman continues, plopping down her bowl. "We can dance. And hanky-pank."

"That causes trouble," the man claims, shaking his long head. "I'm a doctor. I know."

"My father is a doctor," the matron replies. Leaning across the table, she whispers, "He owns the biggest palace in the boneyard."

"Guy walks into the doctor's office," the clownish fool retorts, "says, 'Doc, I've hurt my arm in several places.' 'So,' his doctor says, 'stay outta those places.'"

"How does one leave this place?" John interjects, taking care to speak as if he were talking with colleagues at a conference instead of this collection of witless rustics. "Do you know?"

"There's the door, right over there," the grandam answers, waving a quivering arm.

"I mean forever," John answers, enunciating carefully. "How does one leave for good?"

"For good?" she queries, frowning.

"You die," the jester answers. "Kaput."

Suddenly, the scrawny crone looks up from the photograph in her lap as if she had just woken from a hundred years' sleep. Pushing herself effortlessly upright, she moves slowly between the tables, clutching the photo to her chest like a prayer book or a valentine. When she reaches the weeping woman's seat, she stops.

"There," she says, patting the woman's shoulder. Pressing the photograph into the woman's empty hands, she adds, "There, there,

there." Turning, she shuffles back to her place, leaving the weeper to gaze at the picture in silence.

Now a crew is stacking bowls, gathering napkins, helping the diners to wipe their hands and grunt up from their chairs. Upright, they lurch between the tables and shuffle out the French doors.

"Would you like to go to the TV room for a while?" offers a woman whose bust reads MATTY as she helps herself to John's arm and guides him from the table. "Maybe have a little change of scene?" But before the scene changes, John wants to identify the play. Shaking his head, he leads the way back down the hall, pausing before the open door that leads into a half-familiar room, like a place he's seen once in a dream.

"That's it!" the Matty woman chirps. "You're learning your way around fast. Would you like to take a nap?" she asks as they enter the room and John takes stock of its little bed, plain dresser, and wide window. "Maybe lay down for a while?"

"Lie," John growls.

"Yeah? You want to? Take a little rest?"

But John hates to rest. The rest is silence. There will be time enough to rest hereafter. In the meantime, he has so much work to do that he's joked with Sally he'll have no time to die for centuries to come.

It's the romances he wants to revisit next. As soon as he manages to wend his way out of this strange maze, he plans to immerse himself in their shimmering mysteries yet again.

He thinks they may help in his defense of humanism, though naturally at this stage his ideas are still misty and unformed. But there's something about the way those plays use music, masques, sculpture, and even theater to spark the shift from their tragic beginnings to their joyous resolutions that underscores the old insight that, while tragedy is suffering elevated into art, it's art that helps humans endure—and sometimes even transcend—their suffering.

It's thoughts like that which John wants to give himself to next. He knows he'll need to ponder deeply, to wonder on for months—or even years—before truth makes all things plain. But he's been at this stage in his thinking many times before, when ideas whirl in and flutter on, and insights lead to frustrations that blossom into better realizations. He is certain that if he can only have the time he needs, he will find a way to rescue humanism, even now.

Though the last time he actually tried to read a play, he'd found himself so frustrated by all that he could not quite recall about Helen and Paris and Menelaus and the heroes of the Trojan War, and so puzzled by all he couldn't follow in Ulysses's tangled speeches and Thersites's mocking replies that, after struggling valiantly for half an evening to transmute the words on the page into people and poetry, he finally concluded he'd been reading a corrupted text or maybe even that someone had slipped him a trick copy of the play, like the water-squirting fountain pens or salted sticks of chewing gum his brother used to tease him with.

With a roar, he'd risen from his chair and hurled his copy of *Troilus and Cressida* across the room, terrifying Sally and knocking her great-aunt's mantle clock to the floor. Afterwards he'd been embarrassed and appalled. He hadn't meant to scare his dear love, hadn't meant to destroy her treasured timepiece. But it was such a dastardly prank, not funny in the least, and in the moment he'd been unable to contain his rage.

They'd both been so flustered by the whole episode that after Sally swept up the clock's splintered case and shattered glass, she proposed he might try thinking about the plays instead of reading them, at least for a little while. Especially since he knew them so well, she'd suggested that maybe reading them was only slowing him down.

On the face of it, her idea sounded absurd. But to humor her he'd promised he would consider it, and the more he considered, the more her proposal made a kind of convoluted sense. After all, plays were not a written art form in Shakespeare's time. Not even the actors had copies of an entire script, using rolls of parchment instead—rolls that they called *roles*—on which their lines were written. Despite the exhortations of John Heminge and Henry Condell to *reade him*, Shakespeare had meant his plays to be seen and heard. And what better way to see and hear them—as John had long maintained—but in the theater of the mind? If a play lived inside his head already, why shouldn't he leave the printed version of it behind?

He memorized his first play when he was nineteen, after all.

It's a tale he's recounted many scores of times, a story so permanent in his mind that already the intervening years are dissolving, already that story is washing over him again, already sweeping him out of the meaningless green room where he chafes and waits, and tugging him along on its strengthening current, so that once more he is back in his hometown—or rather, he is in his hometown still—still a lanky, yearning boy, still perched on the concrete step outside the office of Mr. Martini's Esso station, glad that the morning rush is over so that he can take a load off until the next customer comes along.

Holding a Snickers bar in one grease-stained hand and his brand-new Folger's pocket edition of *Romeo and Juliet* in the other, he takes a hefty bite of candy and begins to read:

> *Two households, both alike in dignity;*
> *In fair Verona, where we lay our scene*

Romeo and Juliet is on the recommended reading list for UC Davis's English majors, and John has finished his freshman year determined to change his major from engineering to English.

"And then what?" his father asked on John's first night home while the two of them sat together at one end of the dinner table, their plates filled with the slabs of steak and jumbo baked potatoes that were his dad's idea of a meal to welcome him back. His mother had been dead for over a year, and his last few months at Davis, John had begun to believe he was finally becoming inured to that awful fact, and to think with some relief that, as his father and his brother seemed to have already done, he was honoring his mother's memory by moving on in his own life.

But that first evening home, his loss seemed as raw as ever, her absence searingly evident in the lack of salad or vegetables or even rolls, in the splay of unopened mail that covered what had once been her place at the table, in the carton of salt and the bottle of catsup that sat unabashedly in front of his dad.

Opening a seam in his potato with his knife, his father said, "What on God's green earth do you plan to do with a degree in English?"

"Read," John answered immediately, and although he had not intended to sound so glib, he'd seen how his father's fingers tightened on his knife, how the button of muscle at the top of his jaw twitched just a little. John's brother Herb was already a practicing dentist, had recently purchased a television and a car. "And teach," John added, slicing a bloody ribbon from his steak.

"Teach?" his father echoed. He looked as if the word were a bug that had inadvertently landed on his meat. He had never gone to college himself, and although he'd promised his dying wife he would help their youngest son get his education, he'd always expected that education would help John get somewhere, too.

"Teach," John agreed. Fitting the bite into his mouth, he leaned across the table toward his dad. "At a university," he added, trying to buttress his expression with a confidence he did not own. He had no idea what teaching at a university would entail, but in his freshman English class that spring he'd seen glimmers of a challenge and a solace and a way of thinking that made designing dams and building bridges seem trivial in comparison.

Is now the two hours' traffic of our stage Keeping one ear alert to approaching cars, John finishes the prologue and begins the first scene. Except for the bit of *The Merchant of Venice* he'd inadvertently read back in eighth grade, his experience with William Shakespeare has consisted solely of the play they studied each spring in his high school English classes. His high school teachers' attitudes toward the Bard of Avon have been both precious and pedantic, while the other adults in Kernville seem to consider Shakespeare to be somehow akin to canned spinach or cod liver oil—wholesome and improving, if not always very tasty. As a consequence, John has sensed more than seen the powers those plays possess, their magic having been well-camouflaged by pop quizzes, forced searches for hidden meanings, and class readings whose only redeeming quality were the moments of accidental hilarity they offered, as when, at the end of *Othello*, the kid who'd been laboring over Lodovico's lines, droned, "O bloody period," and the whole class snickered. Or when Eddy Mitchell began Marc Antony's funeral oration by carefully enunciating, "Friends, Romans, countrymen, lend me your rears."

But his English prof at Davis had talked of William Shakespeare as if he were Clark Gable, Winston Churchill, Groucho Marx, and Jesus all combined. *Myriad-minded Shakespeare*, he'd called him, and everything they read, from "On Dover Beach" to *The Grapes of Wrath* seemed to lead back to Shakespeare in one way or another.

The which if you with patient ears attend,
What here shall miss, our toil shall strive to mend.

Romeo and Juliet was the play they read when he was a tenth grader, and John had found it pretty stiff going. He recalls liking raucous Mercutio more than bland Romeo, and he'd been intrigued by Juliet's apparent zeal to lose her maidenhood, since—locker room bluster aside—in his observation, girls seemed more interested in obtaining letter jackets and consuming chocolate sodas than having sex.

Do you bite your thumb at us, sir? Peeling back the wrapper from his brick of candy, John takes another bite. Strands of caramel sag between his mouth and the chocolate bar, and he gives the candy a deft twist to catch the dangling strings. Then, biting, chewing, swallowing, he reads his way down the page, flipping often to the end of the book to consult the glosses, struggling to keep track of which characters are Capulets and which are Montagues, while Hudsons and Austins and Packards lumber by on the street and, from the golden window of the east, the worshipped sun grows warm on his bare forearms.

He is surprised by how alive the first scene seems—much more modern and immediate than he remembers it being in high school. The Capulet servants baiting the Montagues until a brawl ensues reminds him of the fights that sometimes erupt behind the bleachers after the football games. And old Capulet blustering and calling for his sword makes John think of his own father, provoking a smile that is part smirk, part grimace, and part rueful tenderness.

Cast by their grave beseeming ornaments To wield old partisans Though he got an A in sophomore English, he'd actually understood very little of *Romeo and Juliet*. Even now he sometimes gets so tangled in the archaic language and odd syntax that he loses track of who is speaking or what is going on. But it's summer. There are no essays to sweat, no tests to cram for. A feeling of ease floats in the air, a wide warm generosity that seems to hover over Kernville's broad streets and low buildings, spreading out until it includes the river and the endless green orchards that stretch from the city limits toward the vague blue mountains east of town.

He doesn't have to hunt for symbols or hidden meanings, and he soon realizes he doesn't even have to interrupt his reading to look up every unfamiliar word. If he just keeps going, the sense of a line will usually come to him without his having to think about it, in exactly the same way he understands Mrs. Short when she drives up in her '46 Buick and asks him to fill it up and check the oil without his having to stop and define each word she speaks.

A last wisp of breeze teases his pompadour as, waving good-bye to Mrs. Short, he returns to his step and his book. It cost him thirty-five cents, that copy of the play—six cents more than a gallon of gas. He makes seventy-five cents an hour. His fees at UC Davis are eighty-four dollars a year. If he doesn't waste his summer's wages, he won't have to ask his father for much money next fall, a fact he hopes will help to justify his choice of studies.

It did help and it didn't, John muses now while a pair of butterflies spirals around each other like a dancing double helix, for despite his ability to pay his own way through college, despite his scholarships and summa cum laudes, despite all his publications and awards, his father could never quite believe that John hadn't been meant for some other, more comprehensible—or at least more lucrative—career.

But before he can mourn that strand of past too deeply, the butterflies float away, and the sharp, sweet smell of gasoline drifts back across the decades to mix with the algal tang that rises from the river bottom, and John is wafted back to his perch on the station step, lost once more—lost still—in a Verona that is both immediate and mythical, among characters it suddenly seems he knows better than anyone in his hometown.

He has pumped several hundred gallons of gas and his reading step is swathed in afternoon shade by the time the lovers are riddling their way to their first kiss.

> *If I profane with my unworthiest hand*
> *This holy shrine, the gentle sin is this,*
> *My lips, two blushing pilgrims, ready stand*
> *To smooth that rough touch with a tender kiss.*

That youngster knows so little, the John he has become marvels and mourns. That stalwart attendant in his Esso uniform is such a colt. John longs to sit down beside that stripling and explain a thing or two.

About what he might hope for, and what eschew, how best to hew his path through the working-day world.

Or, if the kid refused to listen to John's hard-won wisdom on those topics, at least he might teach him something more about tragedy. Not the simple drivel his teachers had already expounded about hubris and catharsis and how tragic heroes contain the seeds of their own downfall, but other, more interesting insights, like Bradley's observation that it's a sense of squandered potential that makes a sad tale a tragedy, or Frye's idea that the essence of tragedy is the fact that human beings are trapped in time, or even John's own modest discovery that Shakespeare's tragedies ask a third again as many questions as his comedies do.

But the boy on the step does not care about observations, ideas, or questions. He only knows they shine, Romeo's lines. He only knows they provoke in him some welcome hunger, an ache that somehow helps to tame the pain in his heart's core. *Good pilgrim, you do wrong your hand too much*

Later, walking home along the cooling streets, he carries the feeling of those lines inside him. He has left his book at the station, and so can recall only a few scraps of what he read. But as he follows the sidewalks whose cracked and buckled concrete he's known his whole life, he whispers those phrases to the pale sky—*rough touch   tender kiss   sin from my lips*—the words returning to him like remembered flavors or far-off scents, and he feels happy and sad, empty and oddly thrilled, grateful for some unnamed thing that seems even greater than that play.

Exactly as he feels now, remembering.

He begins act two during the midmorning lull the following day, starting with the chorus, and then rejoining Romeo to scale the wall of Juliet's father's orchard and so escape the stale company of his gentle cousin Benvolio and the wild Mercutio.

This time, John finds he is much less enamored of Mercutio,

whose exuberance now strikes him as both more cruel and more crude than when he'd read the play in high school. It is while Mercutio is attempting to conjure Romeo by Rosalind's quivering thigh that it occurs to John that the play contains a great many more references to sex than he remembers from Miss Halverson's English class. A few lines later, when Mercutio suggests, *O that she were an open-arse, thou a pop'rin pear!* the image that leaps into John's mind discomforts him so much he nearly drops the book, appalled that he could imagine Miss Halverson's precious Bard writing anything so rude.

Hurriedly, he flips to the back of the book to consult the glosses, but they fail to elucidate anything. *Open-arse* is listed cryptically as "another name for the medlar," while the definition of *pop'rin* is simply "a Flemish pear." In the end, John decides his own dirty mind must be to blame for misinterpreting Mercutio's line so obscenely.

That summer the smallest thing can twist his thinking back to sex. He thinks of sex when he fits the pump nozzle into the gas tank of Kathy Beecher's Studebaker Coupe. He thinks of sex when his teeth break through the chocolate crust of his Snickers bar or when the river-scented breeze licks his neck. And he begins the balcony scene convinced his mind is so uniquely perverted that he can find sex even in William Shakespeare's plays.

He'd been so innocent that summer, John broods. It wasn't until he studied the tragedies in his junior year that he discovered that *Romeo and Juliet* really did contain the erotic meanings he'd imagined—as well as many more that had not occurred to him. It wasn't until he was in graduate school that he understood that what he'd read in high school was yet another permutation of *Romeo and Juliet's* unobtainable original text, an edition that had been sanitized not by the infamous Mr. Bowdler, but by some other meddlesome do-gooder.

But the John he is that summer has no inkling that the true text of any of Shakespeare's plays is as elusive as the Holy Grail, that every play is a critical and philosophical conundrum that can never be resolved. He has not yet learned about the decades-long controversies over modernizing the spelling and punctuation, nor can he imagine how many hours he will later spend studying articles filled with terms that read like some arcane algebra—*F1, Q4, Compositor X, Sheets C and E. Hand D.*

The boy at the gas station has never even seen any of the plays performed. He does not yet know that the only actors on the Elizabethan stage were male, so that *Romeo and Juliet*'s original audience would have seen two boys standing palm to palm, two boys taking the sin from each other's lips. He hasn't yet read Hazlitt's claim that Romeo is Hamlet in love, or Coleridge's observation that Romeo is in love only with his own idea of love. It will be decades in the future before anyone thinks to explore the homoeroticism in Mercutio's and Romeo's friendship or examine how the patriarchy of Verona adds its oppressive weight to the lovers' tragedy. That summer he only knows that, standing alongside Romeo in Capulet's walled orchard as he and Juliet exchange love's faithful vow, John is at the heart of all that matters most.

For the next few days he lives in thrall, pumping gas, changing tires, and rejoining the lovers whenever he can, following them— through bedchamber, street, and monk's cell—as circumstance and chance tighten around their necks like star-crossed ropes.

Of course, he already knows how the play will end, and yet some part of him keeps hoping he's recalled the ending wrong. He reasons that if he is capable of being so mistaken as to imagine Shakespeare's poetry filled with smut, then it is altogether possible that he might have missed some hidden meaning in the play that will allow the lovers to rise together from their bloodied bier and walk hand in hand into the bright morning of their earthly love. As he nears the final scene, he reads more slowly, searching for the loophole that will let the lovers live, dreading the conclusion he fears he will find instead.

It is nearly closing time on Friday evening when he finishes the play. While he cowers in the Verona churchyard, watching in helpless horror as Romeo drinks the apothecary's poison and Juliet sheaths Romeo's happy dagger in her breast, autos filled with teenagers have already begun to prowl past the station, their headlights and radios blaring in the dusk.

> *For never was a story of more woe*
> *Than this of Juliet and her Romeo.*

After he reads the final couplet, he raises his face towards a sky alive with peach and violet clouds. He feels both flayed and filled, moved to a realm beyond that dusty street, but somehow also connected more deeply to that street, his hometown, and all the world than he has ever been before.

A heron flaps toward the river. Gazing after it, John is struck by the odd thought that Juliet and Romeo are only make-believe. They have never truly lived, not as he is living at that very moment—not so they can feel the little quiver of their meaty hearts inside their aching chests. He knows the same strange comfort he sometimes feels when, gazing into the sky on a cloudless night, he finds himself relieved by his very smallness in proportion to the mystery spread out above him.

But now that he has finished reading it, he also feels oddly bereft. *Go hence*, commands the Prince in the play's last speech, *to have more talk of these sad things.* But in all of Kernville there is no one John can imagine talking to like that.

A Chevy growls by, its windows rolled down and its radio turned up high, a few notes of "All My Love" spilling carelessly out into the evening. Even though John is infamous for his inability to carry a tune, his mind automatically supplies the words to that fragment of song—*I give you all my love.* Long after the car's red taillights have disappeared down the road, the lyrics continue to sound in his head. *The skies may fall, my love, But I will still be true.* Gazing into the darkness where the car has been, it suddenly comes to him that the way he can make sure those star-crossed lovers never leave him is to memorize the play.

At first it seems colossal, impossible, so audacious as to be hardly imaginable. And yet, as he weighs the little paperback in one hand, he reasons that surely it could be done. If an actor can learn Romeo's lines, and an actress Juliet's, why couldn't someone learn both parts—and all the other characters' besides? And why couldn't that someone be him? He has the whole summer, after all, and long hours at the gas station with nothing else to do.

Two households, both alike in dignity He starts in on the prologue as he walks to work on Monday morning. *In fair Verona, where we lay our scene* The air is silvery, sharp as a cramp in his lungs, the light clear and sweet, free of the haze that will thicken it by midday. *From ancient grudge break to new mutiny*

Stopping at every corner, he feeds himself another line. As he walks the next block, he practices the words under his breath, his steps unconsciously limping out the iambic feet. By the time he arrives at the gas station, he can declaim the opening sonnet with hardly a peek at the page. *The which if you with patient ears attend, What here shall miss, our toil shall strive to mend.*

He practices in his head as he pumps gas and wipes windows and counts change. Alone in the bathrooms, while he scrubs the porcelain toilets with Bon Ami, he speaks the words out loud. He likes the resonance the tiled walls lend his voice, and he lingers over his scrubbing to enjoy the sound.

He tackles the first scene during the morning lull. Drudging his way down the page, he repeats each new line until it has worn a path in his mind like the dirt trails he takes to reach the river, and then he tries to find the logic in that line that will help him connect it to the one that follows. When Romeo joins Benvolio onstage, John is grateful for the mnemonics of his couplets—*loving hate* and *first create, breast* and *press'd, sighs* and *eyes*—though the lines strike him as being sillier than he'd found them before, and he hopes he hasn't made a mistake about the greatness of the play.

But he is already in too deep to quit. He finishes the first scene on his way home from work that evening, and day by day the body of words inside his head grows larger, and slowly the play ceases to be a string of lines laid out one after the next, and becomes instead like the spider's web he discovered behind the cash register: brushing a careful finger across one strand sends a shiver through the entire structure, rouses the spider at its center. *Good pilgrim, you do wrong your hand too much   O that I were a glove upon that hand, That I might touch that cheek!   It seems she hangs upon the cheek of night   Go, girl, seek happy nights to happy days   O happy dagger!*

By the end of the summer, he has saved nearly four hundred dollars for college, and, like a child saying his ABCs, he can start at any point in the play and recite his way to the Prince's glooming peace. If he began his project out of love, he has managed to stick with it partly in the same spirit that inspired the greasers in his high school to master the art of removing beer caps with their eye sockets or the frat boys at Davis to learn to set their farts afire. But the longer he works at it, the less his accomplishment seems like a party trick, or even the act of possession he'd first imagined it would be. Instead, it is as if it were he who is possessed, as if the play were growing to own him instead of him owning the play.

Over the years, he learned half a dozen plays by heart—fluently, he liked to claim—and another dozen conversationally. Back in the days before computers, it helped to make his research more efficient. And even after the dawn of searchable texts and electronic concordances, it still impressed his students—undergraduates and graduate students alike—for him to interrupt their laborious paging for a pertinent line by quoting the exact section they were seeking, letting the words roll off his tongue as if he were Romeo or Falstaff or Ophelia. As if he were Shakespeare himself.

Though more and more when he tries to conjure them now, he finds the texts are unreliable, their webs torn, lines dangling unconnected. *idle brain   refuse thy name   'tis gone, 'tis gone, 'tis—*

A crow drops from the sky to land on the lawn like a shiny new thought. John watches as it struts across the greensward, thrusting its black breast forward with each brash step. "Upstart," he mutters, parroting the word the dissolute playwright Robert Greene used to dismiss his rival, William Shakespeare.

There is an upstart Crow, Greene complained as he lay dying in borrowed lodgings, *that with his Tygers hart wrapt in a Players hyde, supposes he is as well able to bombast out a blanke verse as the best of you.* In Elizabethan England, *bombast* meant not only blustering language but also the padding men used to fill out their codpieces. John's students always crow when he shares that fact with them.

He tells his students that William Shakespeare's evolution from an insignificant glover's son residing two days' rough journey from London to a man of the theater that a university wit like Robert Greene might envy is a convergence of miracles that will never adequately be explained. It was a miracle for Will to have survived at all, when two-thirds of the babies born in his parish in 1564 died of the plague before they'd lived a year. And then it was another kind of miracle for a man of William's raw genius and rare sensibilities to have landed in London so soon after the craze for theater swept the entire city, when everyone from apprentices to ambassadors—and even the Queen herself—craved plays, and the first purpose-built theaters were little more than a dozen years old.

John tells his classes that historians can only speculate and scholars only imagine what kind of crisis or opportunity first compelled young Shakespeare to leave his wife and three small children and strike out for London, that city crammed with marvels and horrors, with its palaces and prisons, its cathedral and its Tower, where the river was alive with salmon, swans, and watermen, and the bridge that crossed it was decorated with traitors' heads, that city of lawyers, actors, and bookstores, threaded by streets with names like *Pissing Alley*, *Dead Man's Place*, *Gropecunt Lane*, and *Bear Gardens*.

Bear Gardens, John muses while the crow goes on a-swaggering in the sun—such a blithe title for such a bloody spot—the street named for the bear-baiting arena that was its sole attraction. He has roused many a dull class by explaining how London's early theaters were based on the same roofless, round, three-storied design as its bear-baiting arenas, and describing how Elizabethans loved watching chained bears being set upon by packs of half-wild dogs at least as much as they loved attending brandings, hangings, and plays.

Elizabethan playwrights had no thought of pleasing English teachers when they penned their dramas. Since more than half of the inhabitants of London were barely past adolescence when Shakespeare began to write, John likes to inform his students that a patron at the Globe theater would have been much more likely to be their age than his own. Three thousand people at a time—John marvels as a handful of sparrows scatters across the lawn and the crow cocks his head at some new fancy—three thousand rowdy youngsters crammed inside those wooden Os, the groundlings jostling in the crowded courtyard while their betters preen above them in the galleries, orange sellers, ale merchants, and whores all hawking their wares, everyone gossiping, flirting, and heckling the actors whenever their attention strays from the stage. To hold their audience's attention, to ensure they would come back, an acting troupe had to keep those brawling crowds constantly enthralled.

They were creating something new, John exalts as the crow hops into the air and lofts heavily off into the shining day. Lord Strange's Men, the Admiral's Men, the King's Men—they'd taken a genre that had moldered since its Grecian heyday nearly two thousand years earlier, and they were recasting it to fit their own yearning, teeming age. They were inventing a fresh way to tell a story, a new method to delight, distract, or perhaps even to expand the human soul.

It was a grand collaboration, John rhapsodizes, an unlikely alliance of authors, actors, and audience, all fueled by their desire to push the innovation further, to discover what else it might be possible for a play to say or—

"Dad?"

The voice is timid, tremulous, strangely familiar. John jerks alert with a snort, his speculations scattering like startled birds. But instead of twisting around to glare at his intruder, he keeps his gaze fixed on the scrap of world outside his window, studies the usurping ivy and the peering daffodils in hopes that this interloper will see how busy he is and let him be.

"Can I come in?" the voice persists. He's heard that voice before— or at least he thinks he has—although he cannot at this moment pair it with a name or face. Even so, he feels an unexpected surge of delight to hear it now, though his pleasure is followed instantly by a tug of caution.

"May," he suggests warily.

"Is that okay?"

Reluctantly, wincing at the torment in his hip, John turns in his chair to see a woman standing in the doorway. She is young, twenty-five, maybe, or twenty-seven, a slender woman, all juts and knobs, her brown hair tousled to appear rakish, though at the moment she only seems unkempt, her wafting skirt and sleeveless shirt evidence of the spring weather but perhaps suggestive, too, of something unfixed about her.

She looks eager and worried, breathless in some existential way as she takes a step into the room, reaches out a hand. A second later she steps back to the threshold, retracting her hand to press it against her heart.

"Daddy?" she whispers, her voice catching on itself. Clearing her throat, she repeats more firmly. "Dad?"

When John does not answer, she crosses the floor as if she were wading ever deeper into dark water until she stands in front of him, blocking his view of the windowed world beyond. For a moment she waits, looking down at him, and then she bends into a squat so that she gazes up instead.

Their looks touch. Awareness shivers through him, a complicated swirl of fury and yearning, recognition beyond the provenance of words.

"Dad?" she asks again, her voice wavering before she reaches the end of that short word, breaking it into two syllables, a million questions. "It's been a while," she offers with a small wry smile. "Ten years, I think—come August."

"Ten years?" he echoes cautiously. Her face looks vaguely familiar, though unlike any daughter he's ever known. Whoever she is, she must surely be misprized on that point. Perhaps she is a former student, or a young colleague. Or maybe his bank teller, or the hygienist at his dentist's office. He has met so many people over the course of his travels and his career. Recently he has grown quite skilled at masking his uncertainty about their identities until he can garner the crucial clue that will tell him who they are.

"Do you remember me?" she asks. Her tone seems both beseeching and challenging.

"'I remember thine eyes well enough,'" he says, borrowing lunatic King Lear's reply to eyeless Gloucester as a ploy to buy more time. He

feels pleased to have a visitor who is neither elderly nor officious, glad
to have a guest who appears to have come for the sole purpose of seeing
him. He bestows a smile on her, hoping to win some further hint.

"I'm Randi," she says.

"I beg your pardon?" He tries to temper his surprise so as not to
appear too old or out of date.

"Miranda," she amends. "Your daughter, Miranda."

Miranda, his mind echoes, *Admir'd Miranda,* and, *worth What's
dearest to the world,* and, *my daughter, who Art ignorant of what thou art.*
Despite his inadvertent spurt of hope, he studies her face cautiously,
searching for correspondences and suggestions—her eyes, her lips, her
hair.

"Impossible," he proclaims.

"Impossible?" Her laugh is tight and raw.

Judiciously, he announces, "My daughter has purple hair."

"Purple?" Her hand darts to her head, though a second later her
confusion is replaced by a kind of bemused discomfort. "That's me,
Dad—I mean, it was. I did have purple hair, once, for a little while.
Back when I was a teen."

"Teen," John muses, and when nothing better comes, he adds,
"'Eighty odd years of sorrow have I seen, And each hour's joy wrack'd
with a week of teen.'

"Who's that?" he asks, suddenly sharp as a game show host.

"What?"

"Who says that line?" he prompts, settling grandly back into his
chair to await her answer.

"I'm afraid I can't say who."

"Can you say what play?"

"I really don't have a clue." She is clinging to her smile as though
she fears that she will never find another. "I never really learned my
Shakespeare."

"Your Shakespeare," he tests the phrase. Pausing, he frowns, studies her once more. "Miranda?" he tries.

"Yes, yes." An eagerness brims on her face like water wobbling above the rim of a glass. "Miranda," she agrees. "Your daughter, Miranda—Barb's daughter."

"Barb." He offers the name to his webby mind, gets ashes in return.

"Barb Bradley," the girl urges. "My mother. Your second wife. She moved back to North Carolina. I haven't seen her in a while," she offers stiffly. "But I think she's doing better now. At least she sounds like it, when we talk on the phone."

His eyes travel her features warily, while she waits, brimming. But he's seen that eager, abject look before—on a girl very much like her. And once more it triggers his righteous wrath, once more stirs an indignation so fierce he can hardly fit it into words. "Where have you been?" he barks.

"Me?" She rocks backwards on her heels, throws down a hand to keep from toppling over. "Down in Santa Cruz, the same as always." She looks both frightened and defiant, and he recognizes that irksome expression, too.

"No," he barks. "Previous . . . to presently. Where were you—" He pauses, suddenly tangled in too many tenses, too many *afters* and *befores* and other *nows*, "when you deployed, I mean, departed—when you left?"

"You were the one who left, Dad. Sixteen years ago—when I was ten—you left."

"I?" he asks imperiously.

"You and Mom got a divorce. You moved up to Solano. That's where you met Freya."

"Freya," he echoes, memories assaulting him like petals and hailstones stirred in a spring storm. "She had a fine mind, sharp and . . . keen. But not expansive, not . . . generous. She forgot, that's what she said, forgot to tell me. Though I wondered, later." Staring into some middle distance, he heaves a heavy sigh. "She took the Harvard job."

"I know," Miranda answers evenly. "I mean, I heard."

"It was good, in the end. Riddance. I mean, resolution. She was . . ."

"What?" she prods when it seems he is straying from the path of his own thinking. "What was she, Dad?"

Her question returns him to the room. He studies his visitor, trying to read her hair, her slender arms, the yearning staining her expression. "Why are you here?" he blurts and watches as the yearning stiffens to wariness. "What do you want?"

"Nothing," she answers promptly as a character in a sitcom. Running a hand through her hair, she adds, "Not a thing. I just thought I'd drop by. Sally said you might like to see me."

"Sally," he says more kindly. A long wait later, he adds, "How have you been?"

"Okay," she hesitates for a moment. "Good enough. You know how it is—life, and all."

"I know a little." He nods sagely.

Another silence sags between them. She says, "How about you, Dad? How have you been?" As soon as she asks the question, she looks as if she would wish it back.

"Not well," he answers. "Not well at all. I need to get to work. There's work that needs . . . working on. Important work. My life's work, I might say. We should go," he adds, planting his hands decisively on the arms of his chair and making ready to stand.

"Oh," she blurts, "I'm not really sure."

"I've been here much too long, waiting for—"

"Hey, look," she announces, rummaging in her bag, "I just remembered—I brought you something." She produces a small beribboned box. "Do you still like chocolate?" she asks. When he does not reach to take the box from her, she urges, "I remember you always did."

"I . . ." He hesitates. "Always did."

"Would you like one now?" Untying the ribbon, she lifts the lid, sets the box in his lap. Leaning over to peer at the glossy mounds, she admits, "I'm afraid I don't know what's what."

"None of us do," he answers, taking a chocolate, popping it whole into his mouth, chewing it like bread. "Miranda," he announces after he has swallowed, rolling the word across his tongue like another kind of sweet, tasting the hum and growl and lilt of it.

"What is it you do?" he asks, smiling down at her.

"Do? Me? You mean, for a job?" She teeters in her squat. "I work at a coffee shop."

"I beg your pardon?"

"A coffee shop." She raises her voice slightly. Speaking more slowly, she adds, "I'm manager. I worked up, from barista." She shrugs. "It pays the bills."

"Selling," he breathes in sharply. "Coffee?"

"And coffee drinks." She shrugs, risks an ironic grin. "Espressos, cappuccinos, mochas—it's a big deal these days. There's actually quite a bit to know—origins, roasting times, brewing techniques. All the baristas have their own style—their own philosophy, I guess you could say. It's kind of interesting, actually, but—"

"'There are more things in heaven and earth than are dreamt of in our philosophy.'" He smiles almost dreamily, basking in the line. "'Our,'" he adds with a nod. "That's the Folio talking, and I'd agree. The Quarto's 'your' seems too dismissive—don't you think?—and Horatio is Hamlet's only true friend. They've been students together at Wittenberg, after all." His voice grows in authority as he speaks. "The irony Hamlet's expressing is surely meant to include both of them—*our* philosophy. That's Hamlet's little jab at the limits of their learning, the limits of what any philosophy can uncover, a nod at the mystery beyond."

"I'm afraid you've lost me." She sounds amused.

"I don't remember," John begins, though then he pauses for so long it seems he has forgotten what it was he does not remember.

"Yeah?" she urges cautiously. "What don't you remember?"

"Where you got your degree."

"My degree?" She gives a rueful smile. "I never went to college, Dad—at least, I haven't yet."

"Never?" A surprise bordering on affront sounds in his voice.

"Not yet. I know you'd've wanted me to, but it wasn't a good time. There was too much else going on."

"What," he asks indignantly, "could possibly be more important than an education?"

For a moment she looks stricken. But when she answers, her tone is as pointed as his own. "Stuff," she snaps, though at the sight of his stung expression, she seems to soften, "just a lot of different . . . stuff. Plus, I had no idea what I wanted to study." She pauses as if consulting her thoughts, and when she speaks again, her voice seems to glisten. "But now—guess what? Just two days ago I sent off my app—"

"I thought you might like this," a voice announces from the doorway, and a woman labeled MATTY bustles into the room carrying a straight-backed chair.

"Oh." Miranda rises awkwardly from her squat. "That's nice. Thank you."

"At least it's better than sitting on the ground," Matty answers stoutly, placing the new chair so that it faces the window next to John's.

"'For God's sake let us sit upon the ground,'" John says, his voice growing regal with channeled pain as he watches his visitor settle into her new seat, "'and tell sad stories of the death of kings.'"

"Now, John," Matty admonishes, reaching down to give his shoulder a playful shake, "You shouldn't go talking about sad stories. Especially now that your daughter's here." Turning to Miranda, she adds, "He says the funniest things, your dad. Sometimes they don't make a lick of sense, but other times, they kind of seem to fit. Actually," she continues musingly, "it's that way for most of 'em, really, practically right up to the end. It's amazing what some of 'em will come up with, just out of the blue—sometimes long after you think they'll never talk again. Only the stuff that your dad says," she adds, brightening, "it's different, somehow, like—I don't know—it sounds official. Like it's straight out of the Bible or something."

"It's Shakespeare," Miranda answers. "They're lines from Shakespeare's plays." She makes a self-effacing smirk. "But I'm afraid I couldn't say which ones."

"You're kidding."

"He was a scholar—is, I mean," she says, shooting John a vaguely guilty glance. "Though he's retired now, I guess. He wrote books and taught."

"You mean like *Romeo and Juliet* and stuff?" the stout one marvels. "We read *Romeo and Juliet* in my high school English class. Though if you ask me it wasn't English at all. I was lucky I got a C. Shakespeare," she repeats, shaking her head. "It actually makes more sense when your dad says it than back when I tried to read it. John," she raises her voice as though she could include him in the conversation by yelling. "You never said that stuff was—"

But suddenly she is interrupted by a beeping coming from somewhere inside her bosom. "Oopsie," she says, cramming her hand down the V-neck of her tunic, fumbling between her staunch breasts to pull out a monitor which she glances at briefly before announcing, "Gotta go." As she heads toward the hall, she calls over her shoulder, "Have a nice visit, you two."

"You never asked," John says when she is gone.

He sits in silence, looking out the window. "This isn't easy," he tells the ivied wall.

"It can't be, Dad. I'm sure. I—" she begins, but then she appears to change her mind or lose her nerve.

"Would you like another chocolate?" she asks a long moment later, holding out the box so that it hovers above his lap. When he does not respond, she says, "I'll just leave them on your dresser, okay? Maybe you'll want one later."

Rising from her chair, she crosses the room to place the chocolates beside the framed photograph that is the dresser's sole decoration. "Is this Sally?" she asks, examining the image and then tilting it in John's direction so he can see himself and Sally standing together— Sally in her knit travel skirt, he in his Gucci polo and new dark slacks—the stunning vista of an ancient Greek theater spread out behind them.

"I never met her," she offers carefully. When John still does not respond, she says, "She looks nice."

"I wouldn't say . . ." He frowns. "Nice."

"Really?" After an awkward pause, she asks, "Where was this taken?"

"Sicily. We went . . ." He waves his hand vaguely. "Before." He frowns. "Were you there?"

"No, Dad." Setting the photo back on the dresser, she returns to her seat beside her father. "I've never been to Sicily. In fact, I haven't been out of the country at all—except," she adds after a splinter's hesitation, "for London."

"London—" he echoes. But before he can go further, she rushes to ask, "What was it like, in Sicily?"

"Hot," he answers wearily. "Old."

"Didn't you guys have fun?"

"Guys?"

"You and Sally. Didn't you guys have a good time in Sicily?"

"Guys?" he repeats sternly.

"Oh, right," she says with a laugh. "I guess I'd forgotten. *Guys* is supposed to only mean men."

"From Guy Fawkes. Co-conspirator in the Gunpowder Plot. Contemporary of Shakespeare's," he continues, sitting up straighter in his chair. "Guys were first effigies, then urchins. But always male," he adds warningly.

"Okay, okay." Grinning back at him, she says, "But here's what I always used to wonder: if 'men' is a word that is supposed to include women, then why can't 'guys' include women, too?"

He frowns, thinking. A moment later he shoots her a shrewd, proud look. "I forget where you got your degree."

"I didn't, Dad. I said. There was never a good time. But like I started to tell you, I just sent off my application to Art—"

"We burn daylight." John says abruptly. "It's time to go."

"Go?"

"Leave, depart, vacate this place—hotel," he adds with an impatient flip of his hand, "hostel—hovel—what you will."

"I don't know—"

"I have work to do," he says, rising from his chair. "Important work."

"Yeah, but—I mean, I'm not sure how we can just leave . . ."

"It's easy," he snaps. "How did you get here?"

"I drove," she admits reluctantly.

"So!" he pounces.

"Yeah, but, I don't think—"

"Yeah, but, you don't think," John echoes bitterly. "That's always been the case, hasn't it? That's certainly a theme. Where the hell were you, anyway? Where did you go? You have no idea the doom you caused, running off like that."

"Dad," she pleads, "please, just—"

"I had a chance—a golden chance—but it was mangled beyond repair. And even now, you won't help me do my work."

"I'm sorry, but—"

"Sorry, sorry, sorry," he huffs in disgust. "It's much too late for sorry. Take me with you."

"But I can't just—"

"Take me with you, or get thee gone."

"It's not that eas—"

"Then get thee gone," he thunders, glowering at her as if he might glare her out of existence, "Get thee gone, and dig my grave thyself."

Randi races down the white sidewalk that leads to the back of the building where the receptionist has just informed her there is a smoking area. She moves rapidly, oblivious of the blossom-scented air that enfolded her the moment she pushed the panic bar and burst through the building's front door. Rounding the corner, she walks along a windowless wall until she reaches a pair of stained white plastic chairs flanking an ash receptacle.

She feels a flutter in her sternum, a mounting urgency. Her fingers tremble as she fumbles the package of cigarettes from her bag, takes one out, gropes for her lighter. She runs her thumb across the little wheel, and a flame sprouts obediently. When she inhales, the smoke is harsh and chemical laden, but she lets her eyes slide shut in relief, welcoming the slam of nicotine in her brain, the grateful shudder.

"Good fucking god," she whispers, sinking into one of the chairs while a million emotions battle for space inside her smoke-filled chest. She exhales, takes another drag, then lets the cigarette dangle between two fingers. Gazing at the ivy-covered wall, she attempts to find a shape for what just happened, tries to imagine how she will describe it to Mink, what she will tell their friends, tries to plan the story she will make of it, the few sentences she will use to corral the craziness.

She gives an inadvertent sob, thinking of her father's old, noble face, how his hair had turned completely white since she'd last seen

71

him, thinking how familiar and how strange it was to see him again. Like a dream. She feels a swirl of vertigo, wonders if he will begin to appear in her dreams—now, after all this time. Again.

Three nights ago it seemed like a dream when the landline rang and the woman on the other end asked if she were speaking to Miranda Wilson. She and Mink had been working at opposite ends of the little table that filled their crowded kitchen, he planning curriculum for the summer science program at the junior high school where he taught, and she finishing up the final section of her college application, writing the essay in which prospective game design students were asked to develop a character or describe a world based on one of the images ArtTech College had posted on its website.

It had been yet another revelation, that prompt, such a luscious invitation to do what she was always doing anyway that it seemed almost like a cheat to find it in a college application. The image she'd chosen was a scene of a foggy, craggy world, a place filled with an odd gold light that illuminated distant pinnacles which might be either the spires of an ancient castle or jagged mountain peaks. In the foreground was a lake or bog or calm river in which a creature with features both horse- and wolflike stood, placidly drinking.

She'd named that country Norgone, and when the phone rang, Scrap was curled on her lap like a purring sack of sand, and she was deep into her description of Norgone's history, explaining how generations of greed and disagreement had wasted the promise of both land and people, until all that was left were isolated ragged bands—Dreamers, Warriors, and Farmers—who needed each other's skills and goods to survive, but who looked upon each other with distaste and distrust.

It wasn't the kind of story she ached to make. It was too derivative, too simplistic, too two-dimensional. It wouldn't let a player chew on questions or make discoveries or explore ideas or emotions in the way she dreamed of a game being able to do. But despite all her criticisms, the more she wrote, the more that world wrapped itself around her, pulling her in, inviting her to follow it further, to discover more, proving yet again that, despite her age and sex, despite her poverty and her ignorance of programming, she was right to try to follow this strange calling.

The phone was shredding her concentration with every ring. She cast a hopeful glance at Mink, but the apartment had been hers before it became theirs, and the only calls that ever came in on the landline were for her. Groaning at the intrusion, she cast the cat off her lap, saved her work, and rose to answer. When a voice asked if she were Miranda Wilson, she'd nearly hung up, instantly convinced that only a telemarketer would use her full name, only a telemarketer would ask for her in that brisk professional manner. But she'd hesitated just long enough for the woman to explain that she was John Wilson's wife, and ask if she were speaking to his daughter.

"I would have called sooner," the woman continued once Randi had stammered that yes, her father's name was John Wilson, and yes, he was a professor—or had been—at Solano State. "But I'm afraid it took me this long to find your dad's address book. I've been thinking you should know," she'd paused for the merest sliver of a second, "your father has Alzheimer's."

"Alzheimer's?" Randi echoed. Although she was holding the phone to her ear with both hands, the word slid past her like an eel. Instead, she tried to envision what kind of woman her father's fourth wife was, who he could possibly have found to marry him now, imagining a woman even more self-serving than Freya had been, or even more needy than her mother.

He'd sent a wedding announcement, four or five years ago, back when Mink was just another regular at the coffee shop, a dark-haired scrawny guy who nursed a single coffee for an entire evening while he frowned into a textbook, and who then slipped out at closing time, leaving, more nights than not, a dollar bill folded into a flower or animal or miniature musical instrument at the table where he'd sat.

Her only commitment back then had been to keeping her anxieties and self-loathings contained by making sure her life was small and manageable. She was living in a little dump of an apartment with Scrap, the kitten she'd discovered in the alley one wet night while she was taking out the trash. He'd been a tiny black rag of a thing when she'd found him, with claws like needles and a huge pink mouth, but he'd grown into a sleek, well-muscled creature, her sole ally and her only true friend. His aloofness soothed her, his weight at the foot of her bed helped her to sleep, and if his golden eyes did not exactly read her thoughts, at least they least mirrored them back to her.

She spent her days pulling shots and steaming milk at the coffee shop, and her nights at home with Scrap and her computer, playing her way through one new game after another. *Daggerfall . . . The Ocarina of Time . . . Abe's Oddysee*—she was fascinated by the worlds those games let her explore, the adventures they invited her to embark on. She liked how replenishing her life meter or collecting mana or escaping the Oddworld Stockyard could become such meaningful achievements, and she liked how failing was just an invitation to respawn and try again.

The corny stories, stilted dialogue, and same old epic battles for good and evil sometimes annoyed her, as did the fact that most of the female characters looked like nearly naked Barbie dolls. But there was something about that moment when she first ventured into the caves of Hyrule, or generated a character for *Daggerfall,* or heard that klutzy, cute slave Abe describe his grim discovery at Rupture Farms that made her forget her qualms. There was something about the challenge of learning the rules and figuring out the strategies that would allow her to live and even let her flourish in a new game that kept her both soothed and captivated.

It had been over a year since her mother moved away, five years since she'd last heard from her father, but she recognized his handwriting instantly when the handsome envelope appeared among the usual shuffle of ads and bills in her mail slot. Standing in her apartment's dark entryway, she'd teetered between tearing the envelope open or ripping it to pieces right then and there. Instead she carried it upstairs to her apartment, let it sit on the coffee table like a Hyrulean Bomb Flower that only detonates when it's picked while she checked her messages, fed the cat, and fixed herself a bowl of cereal.

Later, after she and Scrap had both emptied their bowls, she sat in the dusty recliner left by some previous tenant. With Scrap asleep like ballast in her lap, she stared at her name in her father's thin, academic scrawl and tried to imagine what he might be sending her after so many silent years.

They hadn't spoken since her seventeenth birthday, when he'd phoned from some dumb conference or other, trying to pretend that nothing was really wrong, explaining it was Freya's fault he hadn't returned Randi's call when she'd been so desperate to reach him earlier that fall. Of course, she'd realized by then that it was actually lucky he hadn't got back to her when she'd wanted him to. But reaching out to him had been excruciating, and she'd never believed him when he claimed that Freya had forgotten to tell him that she'd called.

She still harbored the vague belief that someday—when the time was right and they both were ready—they would find a way to get back in touch. Once or twice, she'd pondered looking up his number, or maybe even driving up to Solano to drop in on him. But then she recalled how awkward and awful it had been, that time when he'd dropped in on her, and she decided she would wait a while longer.

For the moment, her life seemed just fine in its little way. She was used to her parents being gone. She had her work, her apartment, her PlayStation, and her cat. It made no more sense to revisit her disaster with her dad before she was really ready to deal with it than it did to visit the Fire Temple Dragon before she'd collected the hammer she'd need to fight it. Especially since she couldn't explain the magnitude of her anger without having to tell him things she still could not bring herself to say, in the end it seemed better to just stay away.

Abruptly, she reached across Scrap for the lighter that sat beside her cigarettes on the coffee table. Giving the striking wheel a swift flick, she held the flame poised below the envelope for a long, contemplative moment. Then, as carefully as a surgeon or an artist, she lifted the lighter to run its little fire along the envelope's bottom edge. Slowly the lower corner of the paper began to brown and then to blacken. A corner of the envelope twisted into a curl of ash. Randi watched with a kind of stoic satisfaction as the singe crawled toward her name.

Suddenly a hot orange flame surged up. She felt a spike of panic, an inadvertent dismay. Hastily, she tried to blow the fire out. But blowing only made the blaze expand. She waved the envelope, sending shards of hot ash cascading onto Scrap, who leapt up with a yowl and raced out the open window into the night, leaving Randi to fling the flaming envelope to the floor, and then jump up herself, stomping on the burning paper till she had extinguished all the little sizzling worms of fire.

Snatching up a jacket, she raced out into the dark to scour the neighborhood for Scrap. Hours later, when she finally slumped home alone, the half-burnt envelope lay like a baleful toad on the floor where she'd dropped it. Wearily she picked it up, and when she pried the layers of singed paper apart, she found enough remaining inside for her to read that Jonathon Wilson and Sally Crystal were pleased to announce their marri—

The rest of the engraved message had been burned away. Turning the card over, she discovered that her father had written something on the back. *Sally is*, she made out, and, *I would like . . . if things . . . I don't . . .*

But there wasn't enough of his message left to make any real sense of it, and her more pressing worry was finding Scrap. She spent the next ten days trudging through the neighborhood with an open can of tuna, knocking on doors, calling his name, abandoning the search only when it seemed clear there was nothing more she could do.

Three weeks later, when he finally jumped back through the window while Randi and Mink were sharing a pizza and discussing the potential of massively multiple online role-playing games like *Ultima*, Scrap was as sleek as ever and utterly unconcerned by all the consternation he had caused, and Mink had already progressed from being a gallant cat hunter to becoming a sturdy friend.

By the time she recalled her father's announcement, it seemed like yet another thing best left in the past. She couldn't imagine how she could get in touch with him without admitting she hadn't read what he'd written on the back of the card, and she couldn't think of a way to explain why she hadn't that wouldn't be more awkward than just letting the whole thing go. Someday, she told herself, she would try to see him again, but she wasn't ready—and besides, she was suddenly too busy—right then.

"Or at least some kind of memory loss," his new wife was saying. "They won't know for certain it's Alzheimer's until they do an autopsy."

"He's dead?" Randi gasped, and Mink looked up from his laptop, concern tightening his face.

"He's not dead," Sally answered gently. "But no one's ever recovered from Alzheimer's. I'm afraid it's a terminal disease."

An image of their horrible parting in Heathrow Airport shouldered its way into Randi's mind, when her father had delivered her like a parcel of spoiled goods to the nonstop flight that would return her to California. Freya had not deigned to come with them to the airport, but even so, their good-byes had been excruciating, her father's shame and rage equaling but not mirroring Randi's own. She'd yearned to cling to him, longed to sob out her confusion and her horror with her face pressed against the wales of the dorky corduroy jacket he was wearing. She'd ached to tell him what it had been like, both her adventure and her ordeal, longed for him to help her understand it herself.

When the idea came to her to venture into London on her own, the risk of it never crossed her mind. She'd assumed her dad and Freya would be glad she'd found a way to entertain herself while they were off at their play, and after she'd managed to wander her way to Trafalgar Square, she'd stood at the base of one of the bronze lions, watching the red buses and black cabs circling the wrong way round in the early dusk and imagining how pleased they would be by both her initiative and her accomplishment.

The freshly lit streetlights shone like beacons in the tender gray air, and everything—from the staid stone buildings to the brightly colored buskers—seemed charged with possibility. In that moment she'd truly felt there was no one she would rather be than herself, standing at the heart of that great and ancient city, feeling the thrum of London rise up through her, feeling the world opening out in every direction around her, feeling certain that her own cramped life could change, now that she had seen how much more was possible. Standing in that bustling, balmy, dusky square, she'd understood how small her previous dreams had been.

She'd longed for her father to know what happened next, too, though there was a lot she couldn't really recall, and much of what she did remember confused or disgusted her. She wanted him to help her sort among those splintered memories to find the explanation for what had happened. But she was too embarrassed, still too distraught to try to fit those moments into words.

Even now she feels an inward shudder at the memory of the awful hotel or hostel or dorm room where she'd ended up. Despite all her bravado, she'd been so young. When the room began to spin and a heavy blackness kept threatening to suffocate her, the blond foreign student who'd been so attentive earlier in the evening helped her to lie down, and she'd actually believed even then that he was taking care of her.

"Is nice? You like?" he asked when he began to kiss her, and although it seemed strange to kiss a man so deeply while his friends were in the room, she'd been pleased that he'd asked for her opinion.

And it had been nice—at least at first—and she did like, and besides, she was in a foreign country where, she knew, people did things differently. Even the beer they'd drunk earlier that evening had been different, more like syrup than the stuff she'd tried with her friends that time in Tijuana. In the pub, she'd wanted to match her new acquaintances pint for pint, and they had seemed impressed by her prowess, nodding their heads solemnly and exchanging meaning-laden looks when, at the end of the first round, she'd banged her empty glass down along with theirs.

But sprawled on that spinning bed, she found it hard to remember back that far, impossible to recall whether she'd had another pint or not, impossible to recollect which direction they'd walked when they left the pub, or the buses they'd taken, or the dark streets they'd gone down since, and still the blond man kept kissing her, and still his hands were so insistent on her breasts, suddenly so insinuating between her legs.

She wished he would stop, or at least slow down until they got to know each other better. But she was afraid that if she said so, he might not like her anymore, afraid that his friends would laugh, that they wouldn't help her get back to the hotel. She didn't want to disappoint anyone, didn't want to reveal her own uncertainties, or embarrass herself by sounding like one of those unsophisticated American students that Freya was always ridiculing. And besides, the bed kept tilting so that she had to cling to the man beside her just to keep from falling on the floor.

"It happened so fast," she blurted into the phone, shaking her head to try to clear the memories.

"Not really," Sally answered, her voice so mild it took a second for Randi to register the implication of her words. "They say the average length of time between diagnosis and death is seven years," Sally continued a moment later. "So he's maybe a little more than halfway there—not that I've ever known John to be average," she added with a rueful half-laugh. "He has his good days and his bad days. But in general, it's only getting worse. If you think you'd like to visit him, you probably shouldn't wait too long."

"Visit?" Randi echoed, while a montage of visits with her father played in her head—the corny Disney movies, the awkward dinners at empty pizza parlors, the tense or boring walks along the beach. *Visitations*, her father used to call them, and even at the time it had seemed he was weighting the word with irony, using it to signal all that was forced or flat or wrong about their meetings. But hidden among the false expectations and genuine disappointments, there'd been moments of pleasure or even joy. Brief as the carnival rides they'd taken on the boardwalk, unexpected as the school of dolphins they'd once watched frolicking in the ocean, their pearl-gray flanks shining in the sunset's rosy light, they were memories that moved her even now.

"I couldn't keep him at home any longer," Sally explained. "It got to where it wasn't safe for me to even leave the house. He kept leaving the burners on, or incinerating stuff in the microwave. Once I got home to find the bathtub overflowing. And then, a couple of weeks ago, he was . . . just gone. I had to call the police. They found him eighteen hours later, in the San Francisco public library. It was a nightmare. He had no idea where he was or how he'd gotten there. After that, I didn't have a choice."

I didn't have a choice. Randi heard her father's voice echo down the years, cold with suppressed rage, his voice saying those very words, and adding, *We can't possibly take you to Spain with us now. I've booked a flight to send you home. Pack your things. The cab will be here in an hour.*

"I found a good place," Sally was saying on the other end of the line. "He'll get good care. We're moving him tomorrow. But they say he needs some time to adjust to being there before I go to visit him. Otherwise, he'll just want to come back home with me when I have to leave. They say it will just make his transition harder if I come too soon. It's . . ." Sally interrupted herself with such a quavering sigh that for a moment Randi feared that she was crying. But when she continued speaking, her voice was strong again. "In the meantime, I'm sure he would appreciate some company."

So that's it—Randi thought, suddenly as stiff with resentment as if she were still sixteen—she had finally become useful again, as some company for her father. As though Sally were another character to be developed for her college application, an image of the stepmother she'd never met began to take shape in her mind. She envisioned an enameled woman, dressed and made-up as precisely as Freya had always been, slim and remote and smelling of some expensive, musky perfume, a scent that always caught like a cough in Randi's throat.

"This isn't easy," Sally continued, "but I do have to say that in one way it will be a relief, him being there. I haven't had a full night's sleep in months."

Another memory shot into Randi's awareness—how her father had waited until after the constables closed the door of the hotel suite and the sound of their voices receded down the hall before he turned on her, the fury in his face a thing she'd never seen before, so shocking that for a moment she'd truly thought her real father had somehow been supplanted by an impostor. "I haven't slept for two days," he'd said, his voice coiled tight. "Where the hell have you been?"

She'd yearned to answer him, but she'd been too proud and too ashamed, too aware of her unwashed body and stinking breath to do more than glare back at him. Besides, what could she say? She'd been numb, naive, no doubt still stoned. It was only years later that she'd managed to piece those splinters into a story that explained both her innocence and her culpability.

Sally said, "I know you and your dad haven't been in touch for quite a while, but he still talks about you sometimes. I know he would appreciate a visit."

Why? Randi longed to ask. Instead, she blurted, "Would he know me?" Pressing the phone to her ear with both hands, she tried to force herself into a reality in which her father was both back in her life and so utterly gone, tried to prevent herself from asking what he said when he talked about her. *Still. Sometimes.*

"I'd say there's a good chance he'll recognize you—especially if you go soon. It's not that he doesn't remember anything," Sally went on. "It's more that his memories won't line up. He's still smart. Sometimes he can actually remember quite a bit, especially if it's something he's studied, or something that happened long ago. It's more like he can't keep anything straight, or find the right thought when he needs it. I keep thinking his mind is like a broken necklace—some beads are lost forever while the rest are just scattered everywhere."

A phrase from her late-night studying rose into Randi's mind: *string of pearls,* to describe the kind of narrative that leads to only a single outcome. String of pearls, she'd paused to muse, like the way a story unfolds in a film or a book, where how things happen and the way they fit together is preordained, the pearls arranged according to someone else's plan so that a viewer or a reader is always only an observer, simply moving down the strand one pearl at a time. But video games allowed for other structures, the author explained, complex forms that had yet to be entirely explored—*branching narratives,* he called them, or *amusement park, sandbox,* or *building block* designs, structures that let new stories emerge each time the game was played—stories that even the games' designers might never have imagined.

That's what she wanted to do, she'd thought, lifting her eyes from the screen to gaze at her desires. She wanted to help make the games that would enable those new stories. Computer games were on the cusp of something revolutionary, she was sure of that, with graphics so astounding, worlds so varied, narratives so packed with challenges, heartbreaks, and delights that they would have been unimaginable even a few years before.

There were games set in lands so immense a solo player might literally spend years exploring and still not visit every forest or city—much less each temple, tavern, dungeon, marketplace, or mountaintop—they contained. There were games in which guilds of strangers from real-world backgrounds nearly as varied as their avatars' were—at that very moment—forging lifelong friendships as they embarked on quests in ways no one else had ever envisioned.

But she wanted to take gaming even further. She was convinced that beyond the juvenile dialogue, clunky cut scenes, and silly back stories of even the best new games, a whole new art form was still waiting to emerge, some mix of game playing, role making, and story shaping that had the potential to transform—or even transcend—them all.

That was why she was willing to learn all the math and programming that even the writers on a game team had to know, why she was willing to leave Mink behind in Santa Cruz for four years while she lived in some dull and rainy backwater nearly one thousand miles north, where her peers would be eighteen-year-old nerds and her professors genius geeks who would expect her to work a hundred hours a week.

She couldn't afford it. Tuition alone for a single semester cost nearly what she made in a year, and when she tried to imagine how she would pay for an entire four-year degree, she felt as hot and dizzy and confused as if she'd just been caught breaking some kind of law. But other than

Mink, she had never before been so smitten with anything, never so obsessed that everything she encountered in her daily life seemed only to add to the conversation about that subject that was ongoing in her head.

Not since that triumphant moment when she'd first found Trafalgar Square had she allowed herself to imagine a future larger than her present. She'd survived her father's rejection, her mother's tantrums, and even London and its awful aftermath by keeping herself contained, making sure her goals were near and small. But ever since Mink had convinced her that she should ignore the cost and apply to ArtTech anyway, she'd felt as if she were in a branching narrative of her own. In one way it was as if she were suddenly already freed, no longer simply plodding endlessly toward yet another weekend or puny promotion. But in another way she felt more trapped than ever as she waited to see which version of her future she would get to play—the one in which she could go to college to become the person she wanted to believe she was meant to be, or the one in which that person still languished inside her head.

"It's a little hit and miss," Sally said, "but usually you can still have a conversation with him—or at least part of one—before he gets entirely derailed."

When Randi did not respond, Sally went on, "I know I don't know the whole story about what caused you two to fall out of touch, but I do know that John has been unhappy about it. I can't promise anything, but I'd like to think you might be able to find a way to resolve things, even now."

"I'll think about it," Randi answered more feebly than she would have liked.

"That's all I can ask. But if you do decide to visit him," Sally warned, "you really shouldn't wait too long."

Randi hadn't waited. She'd gone on her next day off. Though now, as her cigarette empties its filigree of smoke into the still hot air, she wishes she hadn't bothered. She'd made her peace with all that confusion and all that pain. Why had she ever thought she should stir that pot again?

"Got a light?"

She jerks from her reverie to see a man approaching down the sidewalk, brandishing an unlit cigarette. His dark hair compressed beneath a hairnet, he wears a large white apron spotted with cooking stains.

"Sure." She finds her lighter, snaps a flame, lifts the pale feather of fire to the cigarette he sets between his lips.

"Thanks," he nods, exhaling a plume of spent smoke.

"No worries."

"It's a warm one," he observes.

Randi nods. *Americano*, she thinks. *Room for cream. Keep the change.* The woman inside—that nurse—she would order something sweet and frothy. A mocha frappe, maybe. Nonfat milk and extra whip. She'd be pleasant enough, though it would never occur to her to leave anything in the tip jar. And her father—what would he drink? A shot of espresso? A vanilla latte? She wonders if she'd ever known him well enough to guess.

"You apply?" the man asks, eying her through the smoke that trails from his cigarette.

"What?"

"For cook's assistant. It'd be my shift," he adds, studying her with friendly curiosity.

"What? Oh no." Exhaling, she shakes her head so that the smoke describes a zigzag in the air in front of her. "I have a job. I wasn't applying for anything."

"Then?"

"I was just visiting." With a toss of her head she indicates the building behind them. "My dad's in there."

"He's a resident?"

She nods. "He moved in a couple days ago."

"Most of the people whose parents are here, they're a lot older than you. I'd of taken you for a granddaughter."

"Nope," she says with clipped forced cheer. "I'm a daughter."

"You okay?" The kindness in his voice threatens to conjure her tears.

"Me? Oh, sure." She gives a brittle laugh. "I mean, it's just a bit of a shock."

"This place isn't so bad. I've seen worse. I've worked at worse," he adds with a knowing roll of his eyes.

"Not the place—my dad. The last time I spent any time around him, he was in London, giving some big speech. And now—" She shrugs, and sighs and shakes her head. In the back of her mind she sees the damp, tamped grounds from a shot of espresso—the puck she has to knock out of the porta filter before she fixes another drink—the flavor and the caffeine all extracted, what's left only good for compost.

Her companion pauses as if to let the weight of her thought settle before he asks, "Now?"

"Now, not so much. I don't know. He really seemed to lose it, near the end."

He nods. "Sometimes they can seem normal or even sort of sharp, and then the next minute they're off in la-la land."

It is exactly the kind of thing she might say herself, though she feels an unexpected resentment to hear her father lumped with "them," to hear a stranger describe him as being in la-la land. But she laughs even so, a tight sharp bark. "He got really pissed when he realized I wasn't going to help him leave."

The laugh that answers hers is genuine, unconstrained. "Wait till he meets Robert. He's been planning to dig his way out for months. Only problem is," he splats his forehead with his free hand as if to shake loose a trapped memory, "no matter how many times he reminds us, none of the staff can ever seem to remember to bring a shovel."

"It's like a prison," Randi says, staring at the wall.

"It's not," he answers. "Believe me."

To me it is a prison, Randi hears a voice saying inside her head. For a moment she wonders where those words came from. They don't seem quite her own, though they fit her thought so naturally.

"Speaking of prisons, you know what they call a telepathic midget who's just escaped from jail?" her smoking partner asks.

"Huh?"

"A small medium at large," he offers, waiting for her grimace and grin before he allows himself to smile. "Robert told me that one."

"Robert?"

"The guy who wants a shovel. He knows loads of jokes, real collector's items, too, from back when he was young. It's fun to swap jokes with him. Plus," he waits a beat, and then adds in a confessional tone, "it's easy to recycle your material."

The smile she offers must not reach all the way to her eyes, because he says, "Lots of stuff's funny in there, if you can find the right angle. I mean," he shrugs easily, "what else're you gonna do?"

Fishing a cell phone from the back pocket of his jeans, he flips it open. Tossing a glance at the screen, he announces, "Break's over. Back to work. Speaking of prisons. It's pizza night tonight.

"What does the Buddha say when he orders a pizza?" He watches for Randi's shrug before he quips, "'Make me one with everything.'

"And what do they tell the Buddha when he pays for his pizza with a hundred dollar bill and then asks for change?" he goes on.

Smiling helplessly, she shakes her head.

"'Change comes from within.' Name's Tony," he says, sticking out his hand. "We'll take good care of your dad, I promise." As he pushes the stub of his cigarette into the dirty sand of the smoking stand, he adds, "See you next time."

After he is gone, Randi stares out over the empty lawn while smoke spirals from the end of her cigarette, and Tony's words echo in her brain. *Next time.* She tries to imagine what another visit might hold that would persuade her to return, but in that moment she can't think of anything. She tried, she thinks. She'd given it one last attempt. Now it's time to cut her losses and get on with her own life. A sickish moisture seems to hover above the green grass, its fragrance an odd mix of chlorophyll and chemical fertilizers. When she stabs her cigarette butt into the sand, she finds an unexpected satisfaction in crushing even that tiny fire.

For the past day or hour or year, John has been watching the little corner of the world he looks out on grow flatter and more subdued while the sky above the wall pales with the waning afternoon. He has been thinking about endings. As the shadows slant toward evening, he has been ruminating on ruin, on waste and costs and casualties, on failure and disgrace.

After his failed address to the International Shakespeare Society, the damage could not be undone, his chance to nudge his profession in a better direction wasted, the final years of his career lamed, his marriage to Freya marred beyond repair, even their European vacation so soured he winces to recall.

He'd never believed that one lecture could single-handedly change the course of criticism, but he'd hoped it would help. He'd known that by arguing for a revival of humanism, he risked being dismissed as soft-hearted and outdated. But after years of seeing William Shakespeare reduced to a function, his plots dismissed as propaganda, and his poetry dissected by tone-deaf semioticians, he had resolved to hazard all for his chance to set things right.

He'd even decided to share some of his own story, in hopes

that by describing how a kid who'd grown up in a community where *Reader's Digest* was considered literature had found himself so astounded by Shakespeare's plays that he'd devoted his life to studying them, he might be able to remind his colleagues about the potential of their profession to affect—and perhaps even transform—people's lives.

It could have worked, he thinks now—and yet again—his remarks might have had a real impact. If only he had slept the night before, if only he'd had the manuscript of his speech on the lectern in front of him, if only he had been able to focus on his message instead of worrying about his wayward daughter. After all, he'd quipped as he adjusted his microphone and looked out across an audience comprised of renowned scholars and their impressionable apprentices, he was speaking to a critical mass.

"*Critical* mass," he'd repeated in hopes of buying a few more seconds in which to gather his splintered thoughts and recall the contents of the speech that was still sitting on the night stand back in his hotel. But instead of the amusement he'd hoped to provoke, the expressions on the faces of his audience appeared to harden ever so slightly.

Ignoring the extra work it already appeared he'd have to win them back, he'd said that, actually, criticism was his subject, the topic on which he wished to speak. It had long been his conviction, he went on, as he focused some corner of his brain on trying to appear relaxed and in control while the rest of his mind surged ahead, straining to recall what he'd planned on saying next, that the primary purpose of criticism was simply to help readers understand—and thus more fully appreciate—a text.

Though it was also true, he'd added, casting a glance toward Freya, who he suddenly realized was sitting beside that hotshot Harvard guy, that understanding some aspect of a text could often help a reader better understand some aspect of the world. He himself had been excited to see how brilliantly the new critical theorists, Derrida, Foucault, Kristeva, and their ilk—their like, he hastily amended—enabled those extraliterary understandings. He had no doubt that the current focus on theory was in many ways making their field more vigorous, more rigorous, and more relevant. But lately he had become aware of some of the limitations he believed those new critical approaches posed, and it was those limitations he wished to address in his remarks.

While his audience sighed and shifted in their seats, he'd gone on to say there were a number of aspects of current thinking that he found worrying. Apologizing because he did not have the exact words in front of him, he reminded them how nearly two centuries earlier William Hazlatt had written that, if we want to see the full force of human genius, we should read Shakespeare, while if we want to see the true failure of human thought, we should study his commentators.

Despite his colleagues' lack of appreciative chuckles, he'd plunged on, offering as a prime example of Hazlitt's words an article he'd recently come across that claimed the very process of failing to comprehend the work of certain important theorists was a significant part of what their work had to offer. Articles like that were nothing but jargon-clotted pseudoscience and sleight of hand, he'd announced, gripping the lectern with both fists as if his conviction alone might convince his audience. Articles like that did justice to neither Shakespeare's readers nor his work. In fact, it was articles like that, John added elegiacally, that were exposing their entire discipline to derision, inviting their own marginalization, driving their most passionate and intelligent students into other fields.

He could offer many more examples of similar absurdities, he'd said, wishing desperately for the manuscript wherein he had listed those absurdities so carefully. He could offer a great number of other reasons for concern, too, though perhaps his concerns were actually linked by a single—and, in his mind, singularly significant—motif, since it was their rejection of humanism that troubled him most deeply.

Humanism, he repeated, groping for the razor-keen phrasing he'd worked for weeks to hone, perhaps the most significant concept to come out of the very Renaissance that had enabled Shakespeare's blooming. Humanism—he'd tried again—that philosophical system that assumes, as William Shakespeare himself must surely have assumed, that all human beings share an essential nature, that, despite such powerful influences as biology, psychology, history, and culture, we still have an ability to exercise free will. Humanism, he continued, leaning toward his colleagues with the zeal of his conviction even as he stumbled over his words, that holds as its core value the belief that human beings can learn and grow and change, and that art—and literature—can fuel that evolution.

But he was so wracked with worry and lack of sleep, his mind so splintered and distract, his tongue so weary and unwieldy that even if he'd had the text of his speech in hand, he would still have been hard-pressed to deliver a stirring address. And the longer he spoke, trying desperately to fill the hour that had previously seemed so short, the more he found himself groping for words or losing himself inside sentences, so that even to his own ears his remarks sounded less like a rigorous and well-considered challenge to the status quo, and more like the sour-grape complaints of a man nearing his retirement—if not his dotage. When he noticed that Freya was not even making an effort to stifle her yawns, he'd had some intimation of the magnitude of his failure.

And thus he botched his best chance. After that speech, he never had another opportunity so golden. The dent that disaster made in his career was anguish enough, but what pains him even more—what still hurts almost past enduring—is the way he failed his whole profession, the way he let William Shakespeare down.

"John," a woman says, barging into his despair like Feste or stone or some other artificial fool, "Has your daughter left already?"

"Daughter?" he echoes, scowling at the raw consternation that word stirs in him.

"That's right," the woman answers. When he shifts around in his seat to look at her, he sees she is carrying a stack of folded bedclothes, which she plops down on the dresser.

"Your daughter," she asks as she peels back the covers on the bed, "has she left?"

"Daughter," John muses, "left." He senses that the woman's question links with the failures he has been pondering, and he offers that verb—*left*—to his fraying mind, waits to see what his mind will give him in return. Snippets of lines float and cluster in his head. *O churl,* Juliet complains when she wakes in the tomb to find Romeo's cup of poison empty, *drunk all, and left no friendly drop To help me after,* while Beatrice confesses to Benedict, *I love you with so much of my heart that none is left to protest,* and Lear's fey fool observes, *thou hast par'd thy wit o' both sides, and left nothing i' th' middle.*

You were the one who left, he hears some other character saying. *Remember? Sixteen years ago, when I was ten, you left.* He feels the same hot instant anger that comes when he accidentally bangs his head or stubs his toe.

"Did you guys have a good visit?" the woman asks, setting a wad of used sheets on the empty chair beside his own.

"Guys," he says, and suddenly the entire visit comes spilling back—Guy Fawkes and coffee and chocolates, an angular, unpurpled daughter. Or at least some changeling claiming to be his daughter, an imputed daughter, though a much different version than any daughter he's ever seen before.

"That's right," the woman nods. "Did you guys have a nice time?" The badge pinned to her bekittened bosom announces MATTY.

"Nice?" he puzzles, turning to frown at her wide rump as she balloons a fresh sheet across the narrow bed. Of all the synonyms he can recall for *nice*—*coy, careful, petty, foolish, precise*, or even *pleasant*—none of them seem to fit either that daughter or that visit, since instead of the reunion he has long yearned for and imagined, a scene of reconciliation to rival the ending of *The Winter's Tale*, it seems their meeting had been a failure, such a disappointment he doubts she could be his true daughter, after all.

Besides, he ruminates as the woman spreads a blanket over the sheets, it was she who left, not he. It was she who left the hotel, she who stayed away all night, she who left him to pass all those hours in panic and confusion. Back home in California, it was she who cursed him and told him to stay away, she who even snubbed his wedding announcement.

His mother left, too.

His mother left one shining morning the spring he turned sixteen, riding away with his father in their black Packard. That was the way those things were done back then, so soon after the Depression and the war. It was a harder simpler time, when a trip to San Francisco was an undertaking, *cancer* a word people lowered their voices to say, and the death of a parent an unfortunate but not uncommon fact of life.

Of course he'd known his mother was ill, but the illusion his family shared was that she would take another trip to San Francisco and come home cured. "We'll be back before you know it," his dad had said, reaching out to clap John's shoulder with his hammy palm as they made ready to go.

His mother was dressed for traveling that last morning, wearing her good wool suit, her best hat and gloves. She wanted to give John a hug good-bye, but he had grown since they'd last embraced, so their hug was an awkward one, she clinging to his shoulders like a dancing partner, while he accidentally bumped her chest so that she'd gasped and winced.

"You're a good boy," she whispered, closing her eyes as if to preserve the moment or to avoid it. "You help your aunt, you hear? I don't want you causing any trouble." Then, her face set in a concrete smile, she'd turned away. Moving stiffly, clutching his father's arm for more than balance, she'd shuffled out to the car and eased herself inside, and when she thought that Johnny wasn't watching, her smile became a cramp of anguish.

He never saw her again. Or rather, he'd seen some poor approximation of her at the funeral, such a meager remnant of his mother in that satin-lined box that at first he'd thought there'd been a mistake or even that someone was playing an awful joke. When, at his father's behest, he'd bent over her coffin to say good-bye, he'd been unprepared for the emotions that battered him. Seeing her lying there in her good suit, her waxen face set in an expression she'd never worn in life, he'd been appalled to feel not sorrow nor tenderness but anger at her helplessness, irritation at the stupid way she'd let her hair be combed, devastation to be confronting such an inhuman thing in the guise of his mother, and terror to think he loved her, even so.

"Suppertime," a woman announces, sweeping into his shadows as pertly as a maid in a restoration comedy. "Are you hungry, John?"

"I don't have time to eat," he answers brusquely. "I have work to do. I need to leave. Presently," he adds for emphasis, and then, recalling what century it is, he amends, "Immediately."

"It's pizza night tonight." Deftly the woman takes his arm and helps him to his feet. "Pepperoni," she coaxes as she waits for him to find his balance. "Mushrooms, olives, sausage—what do you like on your pizza, John?"

"Nothing," he replies, shaking off her hand. "I have to go. I've been waiting . . . all day."

"Eat first, why don't you?" she suggests. "Then you won't be hungry."

In the dining room, he scowls at his fellow diners, cuts a careful sliver from the slice of pizza on his plate. But when he places the tidbit in his mouth, it seems more like some gelatinous cud than anything he can recognize as food. Because he can think of no other acceptable way to empty his mouth, he swallows, reaches for his glass of milk, and takes a tiny sip. The taste of cold milk catches at the back of his throat like sadness. *In sooth, I know not why*

Those were the first words of William Shakespeare's that ever he read: *In sooth, I know not why I am so sad.* It's yet another narrative he knows by heart, part of the story he had crafted so carefully for his ruined speech, and now he welcomes it gladly, happy to leave that sorry dining scene behind and return to a more familiar time instead— some benign, former now in which the plot and themes and conflicts make more sense—an oven-hot afternoon when John trudges into his eighth grade English classroom to discover an unfamiliar teacher sitting behind old Mr. Brown's wide desk, a young woman with fragile wrists and pale hair, perched stiffly beneath the dusty flag with its forty-eight stars.

"Mr. Brown is ill," the substitute announces once the students are all seated at their desks. Her cheeks flushing with heat or perhaps self-consciousness, she asks the class to diagram the sentences she has written on the board, adding that there will be extra credit for anyone who can also diagram the first sentence of the Gettysburg Address correctly.

Diligently, John gets to work, chopping the sentences into phrases and then dividing up the phrases, parceling the words onto their branching lines until he has finished even the final appositive of Abe Lincoln's famous sentence. Setting down his pen, he gazes out the window, watches a buzzard wobble lazy circles in the infinite sky.

"You, in the third row—you need to quit daydreaming and finish your assignment." The other students glance up from their papers, eager for distraction, but when John pulls his gaze from the bird to identify the culprit, he finds the substitute's eyes are fixed on him.

"I have," he answers.

"You've finished? Already?" She holds out her slender hand. "Let me see."

His classmates return to their own thickets of subjects, predicates, and clauses as John navigates his way between desks to pass his paper to the substitute. Red pen circling, she moves down the page. When the pen reaches the end of the assignment without touching down, she gives a careful nod.

"That's good," she announces. "You earned the extra credit, too."

"What should I do now?" he asks.

"Oh," she answers with a little gasp. Snatching up a book nearly at random from the row on Mr. Brown's desk, she presses it into John's hand. "Read this."

As he returns to his desk, he feels a fleeting resentment that he should be given more work for having finished all his sentences correctly. But he generally enjoys reading, and the substitute hasn't said he has to do anything but read. Discarding his discontent, he turns his attention to the book.

It is a small volume sturdily bound with faded red fabric. Lifting the cover releases the heady scent of aged paper, a smell that reminds him of the trunks in his grandmother's attic and the odd old treasures they contain.

The book contains a play, he sees when he flips past the title page. He pauses to peruse a list of unfamiliar names under the strange heading *Dramatis Personae*, but it all makes so little sense that, rather than trying to understand, he turns the page to read the first line of dialogue, which is spoken by a character called Ant. *In sooth, I know not why I am so sad*

And before John can stop to wonder why an ant might speak those words, something is flaring inside him like the fireworks he and his friends set off on the river bank outside of town on midsummer nights. *In sooth, I know not why I am so sad* He has no idea what *sooth* is—or maybe where it is—since it seems to be a thing that one can be in, like San Francisco or a bathtub. But he recognizes what it means, to be sad and know not why. He's felt that more and more of late, sadness saturating him like the morning haze that fills the river bottom in all but the driest weather, sadness lingering like the acrid scent of sulfur long after all the fireworks have been reduced to burned-out, blackened tubes. Sadness squeezing his chest and flooding his throat and heart, even as it rouses him from the doze of daily life. Sadness, with its pang and sting, inviting him to savor more of his existence than he ever had before, back when he was merely a careless kid.

Forgetting the blackboard with its rows of sentences to be flayed, forgetting his brash, dull, or callous classmates, forgetting even the pretty substitute who is sitting now with her hand cradling her neck and her head tucked to one side, he reads the next few lines:

> *It wearies me, you say it wearies you;*
> *But how I caught it, found it, or came by it,*
> *What stuff 'tis made of, whereof it is born,*
> *I am to learn*

It is both comforting and disconcerting to think of sadness as something he might catch or find, like a head cold or a coin. Like Ant, John, too, longs to learn what stuff his sadness is made of, whereof it is born. He keeps reading, the words opening inside him like blossoms, or bombs.

> *And such a want-wit sadness makes of me*
> *That I have much ado to know myself.*

A want-wit—that's what he is, smart enough to diagram the Gettysburg Address, but sometimes so stunned by sadness that he, too, has much ado to know himself. He wonders exactly what that means—*much ado*. And he wonders why it is so hard for a person to know himself.

Recently, in a rare attempt at intimacy, he'd confided to his brother how hard it was to know what he should do or even be. He'd said he could see how he might try to please their dad by trying out for football or joining the baseball team, but it didn't seem like it would be the real John who was doing those things. He'd added that he wondered how he could still be himself if he were to change like that, and he wondered if that other, football-playing John wouldn't also find himself confused about who he was.

"Confused about who you are?" Herb had scoffed when John finished talking. Punching John's shoulder so hard he left a bruise, he said, "You're a person, you germ. Get over it."

The girls in the row in front of him are engaged in a whispered conversation concerning a member of the varsity football team when John turns the book over to read the title embossed on its faded red spine: *The Merchant of Venice*, and the author: William Shakespeare.

Shakespeare—
kick in the rear.

That's the game they used to play at recess back in grade school, one boy ambling innocently alongside another on the playground, and then shooting a foot out to land a blow on the unsuspecting kid's bottom. "Shakespeare, kick in the rear!" the kicking boy would crow, all the while keeping a careful eye out for teachers, who might take exception to that word, *rear*, almost as much as they would object to kicks and dirty shoes.

Back then John hadn't really known what Shakespeare was. Like all the other words whose meanings he'd had yet to learn, it was just a set of sounds with its attendant cluster of apt or outrageous connotations. *Shake. Spear.* To his second-grade thinking, it had made a sort of wicked sense that a kick in the rear would be the outcome of a shaken spear.

But now that he is in junior high, he knows that Shakespeare is one of those famous authors who lived long ago, like Charles Dickens, Jane whatshername, or Edgar Allan Poe. He knows that in high school he will read Shakespeare, just as he knows he will someday study geometry and dissect a frog. Sitting in his eighth grade English class, he feels smug to be reading Shakespeare so soon.

He returns to the play where someone named Sal is talking about argosies and burghers and woven wings, and John is dismayed to find the lines make little sense. Flipping back to the dramatis personae page, he learns that Ant is not an insect at all, but a man named Antonio—a merchant of Venice—and that Sal is Antonio's friend, Salario. One of the salads, John thinks now with an insider's satisfied nod as he recalls how actors refer to those two interchangeable characters, Salario and Solanio, and the boy John was back in his salad days reads what Solanio has to say next,

> *had I such venture forth,*
> *The better part of my affections would*
> *Be with my hopes abroad. I would be still*
> *Plucking grass to know where sits the wind,*
> *Piring in maps for ports and piers and roads;*
> *And every object that might make me fear*
> *Misfortune to my ventures, out of doubt*
> *Would make me sad.*

John has only the dimmest inkling of what Solanio might mean. But he still wants to know why Antonio is so sad, and so he presses on, thinking as he reads how the smallest thing can make him sad—a toy soldier abandoned in a gutter, the curve of a girl's neck beneath her ponytail, the cast of morning sunshine on his bedroom wall, the quiet after dinner.

It seems he is bursting with feelings that need to be shared, questions and ideas that ache to be asked or understood. But still Herb thinks he is a germ, still the other kids in his class are clueless, still the grownups at home are tired, preoccupied with taxes and mortgages and the neighbors' broken fence, and lately, with some new worry that last month caused his parents to make a trip to San Francisco from which they returned laden with gifts for Herb and Johnny, though above their smiles their eyes seemed stark and stricken.

> *I hold the world but as the world, Gratiano,*
> *A stage, where every man must play a part,*
> *And mine a sad one.*

Alone in that crowded classroom, John feels those lines like a kick in the rear, like the suck of some great tide. He hasn't known there are words for what he feels, hasn't known there is anyone who might diagram his sadness, much less that it was William Shakespeare.

But in the next lines, the talk of sadness shifts to debts and loans and suitors, and it is hard to know what to take seriously and what is supposed to be funny. With its chests of gold, silver, and lead, its suitors and its ships, the play seems almost like the fairy tales his grandmother used to tell before she became so old and quiet and confused, though the play is much harder to follow than any fairy tale. Bewildered by the eddies and pauses in the story—Sir Oracle and Sibylla and Jacob's lambs?—John begins to get lost in brambles of language. More and more, the things the characters do or say make no sense. Why would Antonio agree to lend Bassanio money he doesn't actually have? Why would Shylock let Antonio borrow money without interest when he dislikes Antonio so much? What makes Portia such a prize? Why is it so bad to be a Jew?

As far as he knows, John has never met a Jew, though he's stared at the photographs of the concentration camps in *Life* magazine, studied the twig limbs of the living and the cordwood piles of the dead and felt that awful shiver of horror, the fascination and perplexing complicity of a survivor. He is not quite sure what it means, to be a Jew, though he is generally grateful he does not have to be one. But when he learns that Antonio has spat on Shylock even before the play began, he feels a sudden deep connection with the man all the other characters call the Jew. Later, when Antonio admits he is likely to spit on Shylock again, John finds his sympathies skewed unexpectedly away from the merchant of Venice, and he wonders what part of the story he has misunderstood.

Not much, the newer, older John muses while his milk sits undrunk and the pizza on his plate congeals. He feels a paternal tenderness for both the ardor and the melancholy of that former self, feels a wash of pride for the innocent astuteness of his response to that troublesome play. He wishes he could have had that boy as a student. He could have done a lot with a kid like that.

Supper over, he is returned to his cell to find that someone has turned the lights on so the room's interior is brighter than the gloaming outside. When John resumes his chair, he meets a faint image of himself hovering on the window glass, his own worried face separating him from the dimming world beyond.

And in a trice, time shifts so that he is facing another darkened window—the window in the little sitting room of their suite in the hotel off King's Road—where he stares at another troubled version of his reflection. Furious and worried, seething with tension and trying to stay calm, he asks that dark reflection what he should do. It is two o'clock in the morning, or maybe three, but he has not yet been to bed. The air is saturated with the scent of the vast bouquet of lilies that the International Shakespeare Society sent to welcome him to London, though now the flowers' swoony reek only adds to his unease.

When he lifts the window sash, a breeze sweeps the stuffy room. Leaning out into the night, he inhales until his lungs lurch from the effort, while he scans the street four stories below. But the only people he spies are a pair of late-night revelers stumbling along the pavement arm in arm. Even from that distance, it's clear that neither of them is his errant daughter.

He has no idea how alarmed he should be. He only knows that three hours earlier, as he and Freya were returning to the hotel from seeing *As You Like It* at the Barbican, he'd felt more sanguine than he had in months—so pleased about the present and optimistic for the future that, like the Constable landscapes they'd admired in the Tate Britain earlier that day, even the past seemed to have taken on a rosy glow.

Three hours ago, he'd been eager for the coming morning, when he is scheduled to give the opening address at the ISS's annual conference. He has an urgent message to share, one he believes with his whole heart, and which he hopes will do at least its small part in restoring sanity and significance to his profession. He has worked all summer on his plea for humanism, has worked harder than he has ever worked on anything before, but now when he imagines delivering that speech in less than six hours' time, it seems more ordeal than opportunity, since he knows that even if Miranda were to reappear at that very moment, it is already much too late for him to get the rest he needs to be his keenest on the morrow.

Earlier that evening, he'd believed their trip was playing out well. He'd felt confident about the conference, and he'd also been hopeful that by the time their travels in England and Spain were over, Freya, Miranda, and he would have finally succeeded in fashioning a viable family out of the odd triangle of the three of them.

Freya had made it clear from the start that she had no interest in children of her own, and at first John had seen that as a good thing, since it meant Miranda would never risk being marginalized by a second family. Later, he'd come to realize that if mothering her own theoretical children did not appeal to Freya, mothering any actual children of his held even less attraction for her.

But Miranda had a mother. What she needed was a role model, and Freya was brilliant, determined, fiercely resourceful. Her own mother had died at thirty, her father wore dentures from the age of thirty-four, and none of her seven siblings had graduated from high school, while Freya had managed to win so many scholarships and grants that by the time she received her PhD, she had $20,000 in the bank. John hoped Freya's drive would prove an antidote for Miranda to her mother's indolence, that Freya's intelligence would help Miranda learn to value intellectual pursuits.

Over the last half year or so, he'd seen signs that Miranda and Freya were beginning to appreciate each other, with the two of them connecting over the most unexpected things—horror films, and hedgehogs, and anchovies on their pizzas. When John proposed that Miranda join them in Europe, Freya's only stipulation had been that she would need to have her own hotel room.

They'd had some rocky moments, to be sure, beginning when he and Freya arrived to bring Miranda to the airport, only to be confronted by the spectacle of her three huge suitcases and her newly dyed hair. But he'd managed to soothe and smooth and tease and cajole until both Miranda and Freya, and finally even Barb, had graced him—if not each other—with grudging smiles.

Later, in the San Francisco airport, while Miranda wandered off to stock up on magazines and candy for the flight, John had made light of her latest fashion decisions to Freya. Hair would grow, he'd assured his well-coifed wife, dye would fade, and he had no doubt that Europe had welcomed many a lavender-headed hoyden before Miranda. He'd even managed to provoke a laugh from Freya, when, misquoting Benedick's thoughts on the necessity of procreation in his *I did never think to marry* speech in *Much Ado*, he'd punned, "The world must be purpled."

On their ride in from Heathrow, Freya had taken the cab's backwards-facing bench so that Miranda could enjoy the better view.

Angling her lovely calves beneath the seat, she'd promised Miranda that the two of them would visit Madame Tussauds together, archly informing John that she expected those wax replicas of celebrities and murderers would offer her an excellent analogy to use in her next article on signs and signifiers.

Naturally, he was disappointed when Miranda announced she had no interest in attending *As You Like It*. But he wanted her to see he respected her agency, hoped she would learn to appreciate literature and the theater on her own terms and not just at his behest. Besides, he'd had to admit that an evening at the theater with Freya alone had its appeal. They had each been so focused on their own work that summer. Now he was looking forward to reviving their amour.

Miranda's note was waiting on the table in their sitting room when they returned from the play. Her jet lag was keeping her from sleeping, she'd written, so she'd gone out for a little walk. She would be back soon. She'd signed her message, *love randi*. It was the first time John had ever known Miranda to butcher her name like that, and along with his annoyance at the lack of a comma and the lowercase *r*, he'd made a mental note he needed to warn her how "randy" would be interpreted in England.

He was more than slightly irked that she had not understood how foolish it was to traipse off on her own in a strange city at night, and he assured Freya that as soon as his speech was over, he and Miranda would have another chat about rules and expectations.

"She won't be long," he promised with a kiss that augured finer pleasures to come. "She'll be back before you get your makeup off."

But that had been three hours ago. Since then, Freya had taken a bath and done her nails, and, when Miranda still had not appeared, she'd opted for flannel pajamas instead of the negligee John had given her as a travel gift and gone next door to sleep while John waited in the sitting room to greet his wayward daughter.

Now, as the tardy-gaited couple disappears around the corner, John imbibes another draught of chill city air and tries to decide what he should do next. He's already searched the hotel lobby and the bar. He made a round of nearby pubs only to find them closed. He interrogated the night clerk, who claimed to have noticed no lone young women during his shift, and certainly none with purple hair.

The clerk offered to contact the police, but John had been alarmed by that suggestion. Miranda was nearly seventeen, after all. For better and worse, being raised by her mother for the last six years had made her independent. Despite her miscalculation this evening, he still believes she is relatively streetwise. He doesn't want to risk their relationship by inviting the London police force into it, doesn't want to cause a scene where none is warranted—especially not in a foreign country, especially not when he has to give the most important speech of his career in six hours' time.

Uneasiness growing in his belly like a tumor, he lowers the window and snatches up the phone. But when he hears the foreign dial tone spiraling from the earpiece, he replaces it in its heavy black receiver. As he returns to the window to scan the dark street one more time, a familiar round of questions begins to grind inside his head: maybe there was more he could have done for Miranda in these last few years, perhaps he should have suggested a change in the custody arrangements, or even offered to send her to a boarding school.

But now—and yet again—the counterarguments begin, since he hadn't wanted to destroy Miranda's equilibrium, fuel Barb's resentments, or add extra stresses to his new marriage by proposing any changes prematurely. And in the meantime, hasn't he done everything he could? He's attended every school performance and teacher conference, padded his support payments with extra money for dance lessons and braces. He's insisted on keeping up their regular schedule of visits despite all the commitments, distractions, and enticements in both his and Miranda's lives of late.

Lowering the window, he stares into the eyes of his reflection while his thoughts return to the performance of *As You Like It* he and Freya had attended earlier that evening—the kindly Duke Senior celebrating his sweet life in the Forest of Arden while his daughter Rosalind relies on her native judgment and sparkling wit to conjure her own path through the working-day world. Of course John understands that a comedy is no recipe for living, and yet beneath its charming surface, *As You Like It* is laced with so many kinds of wisdom. When Duke Senior's cruel brother tries to control his own daughter by commanding that she give up her friendship with Rosalind, Celia defies her father and runs away from home.

But Duke Frederick is a tyrant, John thinks, tearing himself from his memory of that night as if escaping an incubus. Frowning at the dark, lined countenance frowning back at him, he attempts to follow his thoughts about Shakespeare's fathers and daughters further. Yet, although he can list many examples of miserable daughters—Juliet, Ophelia, Cordelia, and Hermia, to name just a few—tonight it strikes him that the merriest maidens in Shakespeare's plays—Beatrice, Viola, Perdita, Rosalind, and the like—are those whose fathers have little or no presence in their lives.

But instead of harping on daughters, John finds his thoughts harking back to London, where once more he sees the black helmets and stubby billy clubs of the pair of constables he finally asked the clerk to summon not long before dawn, once more cringes at their supercilious manners, once more feels how surreal it seems to try to explain to those two strangers why he and Freya left Miranda alone all evening, why they did not call the authorities the second they realized she was gone.

Once again he feels the prickle and twist of escalating anxiety as the city starts to brighten with the coming day, the time for his speech draws nearer, and still there is no sign of his daughter. Once more he tries to calculate to the second how long he can afford to wait for Miranda at the hotel and still make it to the conference on time, once more hears Freya's hot rebuttal when he suggests she might stay behind in hopes of Miranda's returning while he hurries on ahead. It won't change anything, Freya counters, if neither of them is at the hotel when Miranda comes back; in fact, it might even do Miranda some good to realize that other people have lives, too. And if—as Freya severely doubts—something bad really has come from his daughter's latest escapade, then Freya's waiting at the hotel won't change that, either. Miranda's fate is out of their hands, and this conference, as Freya sourly reminds him, is at least as important for her career as it is for his.

Now he recalls how Freya's annoyance ices the boxy taxi as they race down the Embankment towards the college, remembers how she crosses her legs and turns her head to glare out the window at the gray river they'd admired so contentedly from their Bankside restaurant the night before. When they arrive at the conference site at last, he leans across the miles of the cab seat to render her a kiss she winces to receive. Then he is thrusting a rough bouquet of banknotes at the cabby, then running down an endless marble hallway with a conference official trotting at his side, the flustered woman trying to assure both of them that everything will turn out brilliantly, while he apologizes for his tardiness and strains to camouflage his burgeoning consternation because it has just occurred to him that, amidst all the morning's panics and confusions, he has left the text of his speech back in their hotel room.

He can see it there, as he jogs beside the breathless official—that little stack of pages waiting innocently next to his bed, his entire summer's work summed up so succinctly, the key to all he wants urgently to impart.

As they sprint down the final hall, he tries to convince himself he doesn't need his written-out speech. He knows what he wants to say, and nothing flattens the passion of a talk more than reading it. He reminds himself that in his classes, his best lectures are always the spontaneous ones, when he adds his students' growing interest to his own enthusiasm and then rides the rising wave of that excitement to reach some thrilling new shore. He can do that now, he exhorts himself. He has both the passion and the knowledge to deliver his best speech extempore.

Then he is standing in the wings of the lecture hall stage as the president of the International Shakespeare Society embarks on her introductory remarks. Teetering between worry and fury, he tries not to imagine where Miranda is at that very minute, tries not to imagine what she might be doing—or what might be being done to her—tries to convince himself that, despite his missing manuscript and the disaster of the last few hours, his lecture can still be the success he hungers for it to be. He tries to ignore the grim epiphany he has just had in the hallway, that although it is still more than likely that Miranda will turn out to be just fine, the damage she has already caused him may never be undone.

"Bedtime," a soft voice announces. "Mistah Wilson, it is time for bed." A delicate, dark woman slips into the room. John watches her progress in the black mirror of the window as she takes a pair of pajamas from the dresser, sets them atop the little bed. "Put dese on, please," she says, her accent musical, her diction enchantingly precise, "and I shall return to help you wit your teeth."

"Wherefore?" John growls, twisting around in his chair to scowl at her.

"I beg your pardon?"

He makes a small disgusted wave in the direction of the pajamas.

"It's time for bed," she answers simply. The badge on her slight front reads ELIZABETH.

"It's time," John replies regally, "to leave. I've been waiting all day."

"You have had a long day," she agrees as she eases him to his feet.

"There's been a mistake. I don't belong here. I need to leave."

"You will soon become accustomed to it here."

"Who's in charge? I need to speak with whomever is in charge."

"Ms. Michaels is de name of our director. But I fear she is not here dis time of night. Perhaps you may speak wit her tomorrow."

Frustration boils up in John like hot pitch. But he sees he is caught in a seamless trap. He can't make his true needs known, can't find a way to hold anyone accountable. There are too many motifs, too many ambiguities he can't interpret. Any kind of scene will only make things worse. In a slash of revelation, he understands that he can demand to see Ms. Michaels all he wants. But at this petty pace, tomorrow will never come.

"Put on your pajamas," the woman urges. "And I shall return to help you wit your teeth."

And then she is gone, leaving John to glare at the foolish pajamas. With their dark blue piping and the tangle of monogram embroidered on the useless chest pocket, they might almost be called handsome. But he hasn't worn pajamas since he was a child, instead preferring to sleep nude, either luxuriously alone between smooth sheets, or pressed luxuriously against another's flesh.

He is lonely, suddenly utterly lonely, entirely alone inside his own sad skin, alone in a sorry life he does not recognize, alone in a graceless room, attended by a stranger who wants him to put on his pajamas. He yearns for someone who knows him, for anyone who can tell him who he is. He wants his life back, his right and righteous life. His real life, rife with true tomorrows, rich with mornings and evenings and afternoons. Not this endless empty existence in this institutional room.

"Oh, Mistah Wilson," a woman remonstrates, nudging him from

his sorry reverie. She stands in the open doorway, her slender arms akimbo. The badge pinned to her blue tunic proclaims ELIZABETH.

She leads him toward the bed where the foolish bedclothes lie. Planting herself beside him, she waits until it seems he has no choice but to shuffle off his slacks and shirt and stagger into the pajamas. He feels doltish, frustrated as a child as he attempts to get the tubes of fabric to correspond to his stiff limbs. Twice he has to pull the bottoms off and start again. But finally he stands in the middle of the room, his pajamas on, his hands hanging empty by his sides.

"And now, your teeth," the woman urges, trundling him into the bathroom, offering him a toothbrush. After he has scrubbed and spat, she escorts him back to the narrow bed, helps him to climb between the bleachy sheets.

"Shall I close de curtains?" she asks, moving toward the window and reaching for the wand to pull them shut. But John waves a curt refusal in the air.

"All right," she cedes quietly. Crossing to the open doorway, she switches off the light. "Good night," she says as she slips out of the room, leaves John lying like a corpse beneath the bedcovers.

Cautiously, he turns his head so he can look out the window, trying to discern the creeping burglars or looming monsters, the newts and blindworms, or secret, black and midnight hags lurking for him out there. But he can make out only the lacy silhouette of a tree, a denser darkness beyond. It's inside where the demons live, in the regrets he cannot conquer, the grievances he cannot overcome.

Who's there?

That's how *Hamlet* begins, with a sentinel's brief challenge at the midnight changing of the guard. It's such a simple opening that semester after semester John's students race right past it. And semester after semester he has to slow them down, to send them back to the beginning to ponder that question more deeply.

But tonight, as he lies waiting in the dark for death or morning, he wonders if he's ever really pondered that question for himself. Surely he has, he thinks—he must. And yet it seems another thing he has forgotten, another fact that's drifted off, another shred of understanding lost in the mortal shuffle.

Inside his chest, the meaty engine of his heart thuds out an answer of its own. He can feel it even now, pumping out the primal iamb of his existence—*I am, I am, I am, I am, I am*—tapping out his life's long sentence.

The sentence that sentences him to dust: *I am.*

But who?

How can he have lived so long and still not know?

He's in a room. He's sitting in an anonymous green bedchamber, gazing through clear glass at a plot of grass imprisoned by a tall brick wall. Ivy festoons the wall, and a row of rose bushes lines its base—crimson, saffron, and ivory roses in full midsummer bloom. John studies that strange garden by the hour, the grass, the bricks and ivy, the roses and the breezes and the passing butterflies.

He's in a room, but not his own. Though they lie and tell him that it is. Strangers come and say they want him to be comfortable, ask if there is anything he needs. And then don't wait to hear his answer, don't stop to question what he means when he barks, "O, reason not the need," or pleads, "I must needs be gone." Instead they smile and smile and smile. Instead they pat his shoulder as if he were a toothless dog or a sun-warmed stone, and hurry off to other things, leave him alone.

Alone, like to a lonely dragon.

But that was Coriolanus, exiled from Rome. And he is John—Professor Wilson—exiled from his work and wife and home. He is Dr. Wilson, abandoned like a burned-out chimera in this strange green room.

In theater parlance, a green room is where actors pass the time when they are not performing. Like a decompression chamber, like limbo or purgatory, a green room is a place between, a place where, costumed and ready for the stage, players await that alchemical moment when they shed their other selves and join the play. There was a green room at Blackfriars Theater, John recalls with a burst of pleasure as if welcoming a visitation from a long-absent friend—though in *A Midsummer Night's Dream* when Peter Quince's troupe of rude mechanicals gathers in the woods beyond Athens's walls to rehearse their play, they call it a tiring house instead.

This green plot shall be our stage, Quince claims, *this hawthorn brake our tiring-house.* And it's in that makeshift green room that Bottom gets translated, changed from a stagestruck weaver to the donkey-headed lover of the fairy queen.

Changed in a green room in a green world! John epiphanizes. He wonders if he's had—or maybe read—that thought before, or if it's as fresh an insight as it suddenly seems to be. Either way, it pleases him inordinately, to think that the most magic moment in that most magical of plays would occur in such a twice-enchanted place—a green room in a green world.

Green worlds, he thinks with a satisfaction as deep as if he had just taken the first taste of a full-throated, peaty scotch. Settling back into his chair, he lets thoughts about green worlds roll through his mind, savoring that moment of apprehension, the feeling that he is once more in command. Green worlds, he mulls, teasing out the flavors—those luminous, liminal, verdant places where characters are drawn—or maybe even driven—to escape harsh laws, or cruel fathers, or some other wreckage in their working day lives.

Green worlds, John continues with a scholarly nod at the assembled roses, those forests, islands, or distant coasts—Arden, say, or Bohemia, or Illyria, or Prospero's enchanted isle—where everything is topsy-turvy and the normal rules do not apply, where enlightenment comes by way of confusion, where men and women must lose themselves entirely to find themselves anew.

Changed in a green room in a green world, John rhapsodizes. It's a thought he yearns to share with Sally. Gazing out upon the bee-kissed roses, he smiles, imagining her pleasure when he tells her. *Dream* is one of her favorite plays.

Sally has been to see him. He suddenly recalls.

Somehow she managed to find him, even stranded as he is in this desert place. Sally, his last, best, dearest wife. Sally, his soul's solace and his life's delight, the wife with beauty in her eye, since, as he is fond of telling her, beauty is in the eye of the bee holder.

She'd worn a dress he did not remember ever having seen her in before, her hair was arranged in some new way, and she seemed so nervous and slightly strange that at first he hardly knew her. Though even before he'd named her and claimed her as his own, his spirits had leapt up at the sight of her as if he were a mere boy, a green, untutored youth glimpsing the lass to whom he had just lost his fresh-minted heart.

She brought with her a whiff of the world beyond, a scent of purpose and busyness, a casual wide freedom he'd nearly forgotten one might possess, the great reckless bounty of the ordinary everyday. He held her for a long time. Eyes closed, standing in that meager chamber they kept insisting was his, he'd pressed his Sally against his chest, inhaling the faint scent of honey that never seemed to leave her hair, and beneath that, her own dear private smell, while he nearly swooned with his longing to merge with her—not just his little tongue or soft old penis, but his entire self commingled and subsumed.

"How are you?" she'd whispered into his chest. But that was a question past the wit of man to say, and so he'd shook his head, buried his face deeper in her sweet honey hair, breathed her in and in and in.

"I've missed you," she whispered. Into the quiet that followed, he'd strained to find something he could say to fit all that he was feeling, but in the end he could only nod and say, "Okay."

She sat beside him and held his hand, the two of them gazing out the window as if they were attending a play together—watching the rising action of a pair of butterflies, the denouement of a passing squirrel. She asked him about himself, but when he could not muster an adequate reply, she began to cram the air with news of queens and drones and nectar flows, of splitting hives and catching swarms and fixing the extractor.

After her talk dribbled to an end, he'd offered, "You are my—" But his throat squeezed shut before they could find out what.

She sat with him until the color had leached from the scarlet and yellow roses, leaving the white ones glowing like sweet sorrows in the graying air, and when she said she had to go, he'd sprung up, too. "Oh, John," she answered, her voice raw with pain. "You've got to stay."

"Please," he'd blurted. "I can't . . . bear it." He'd hated to have to plead his case, hated to reveal how utter his desperation was, hated to have to burden her with him. But even worse than all those hates was the moment that came after, as he watched the pain on her face harden into the same resolve he'd once spied in her expression when the cat dropped a rumpled starling on their doorstep, and rather than allowing the creature to suffer any further, she'd smacked the life from its broken body with the back of her shovel blade.

Sally's visit was yesterday. Or the day before. Or any day but this one in this odd unjointed time. Today Sally is gone, and John is bearing it still—still chained to his stake and trying to hold his ground while the growling curs ring him round, still fighting the course that will end in only one way, since no bear can live forever with a chain around its neck.

From behind him comes a sound like the near words of a stream, or perhaps the *rhubarb, rhubarb, rhubarb* actors learn to murmur during crowd scenes to mimic background talk. Groaning around in his chair, John discovers yet another mooncalf barging into his room, this one a scarecrow who walks with his head bowed nearly to his chest, muttering as he comes.

"Vanish," John growls, waving toward the door. "Depart. Beat it hence."

But the dotard marks him not. When he reaches the window, he stops, gazes at the verdant walled world beyond.

"That tuna was bigger than Methuselah," he interrupts his gabbling to announce. He taps the glass with his forefinger. "This melts when it rains. Did you dress warm?"

"Warmly," John snaps.

"Sez you," the man replies. "Goddamn you anyway, you motherfucking whore." He gives the pane a resounding slap with the flat of his palm.

"Shog off, elf-skin," John snarls. "Go fill some other grave." At last the clodpoll turns and drumbles off, babbling as he goes.

A' babbled of green fields. That's what Mistress Quickly says when she describes the death of her irksome friend and favorite customer, Jack Falstaff. Or at least, John recalls with a satisfied nod at the squirrel that dashes across the lawn like a brief silk scarf, that's how Falstaff dies according to Lewis Theobald's emendation. *And a Table of greene fields* is what's printed in the Folio, making it a stretch that Shakespeare himself ever intended *babbled.* But whatever Shakespeare actually meant is lost in the vapors of time, and although Theobald was no poet—although he plagiarized another man's play and provoked Pope to write him down a dunce—as an editor of Shakespeare, he was both thorough and inspired.

And how can Falstaff not die babbling, John wonders as the lack-brain blabs his way on down the hall—especially after nearly three hundred years of its being so? As he's oft explained to students, the most a modern editor can do is gloss the matter, offering up a footnote's worth of history and a quibble's worth of question before leaving the fat knight to find his way to Arthur's bosom according to Theobald's emendation.

But rather than musing on emendations, John finds himself succumbing to Falstaff's gravitational tug. Not the faux Falstaff of *The Merry Wives of Windsor*—the foolish buffoon in that fatuous play that legend has it Shakespeare knocked off in a fortnight because Queen Elizabeth wished to see fat Jack in love—but the real, raw rogue himself, the Falstaff of the Henry plays, Prince Hal's friend, Mistress Quickly's sometime lover, Boar's Head Tavern's greatest philosopher.

Jack Falstaff, John thinks fondly, one of Shakespeare's roundest characters—next to bony Hamlet, bonny Rosalind, howling Lear, and leering Macbeth. Sweet Sir Jack, who is born an old man with a white head and a round belly, and who dies a child, playing with flowers and smiling upon his fingers' ends. True Jack Falstaff, John eulogizes, that great waxing moon of a man compared to Prince Hal's lean imitation sun.

When the squirrel reaches the base of the tree, it jerks to a stop, studies its surroundings in tense little starts like a film being shown one frame at a time. Then, defying gravity, it flows up the trunk, vanishing among the shiny leaves. Long after the tip of its feathery tail has disappeared, the shadows on the ground tremble with remembrance of its passing, while John's mind trembles with images and broken lines. *God send the companion a better prince!* *We have heard the chimes at midnight* *I was now a coward on instinct* *banish plump Jack, and banish all the world*

Gazing at the unsquirreled tree, John recalls the first Falstaff that e'er he saw—a jolly, pillow-enhanced version—rollicking with Prince Hal and Poins in *Henry IV, Part I*. His attendance at that performance is yet another tale engraved upon his heart, another saga from his stored and storied past, and he embarks on it now, grateful for the respite waiting for him at UC Davis more than half a century ago—back when it was his time to play a yearning undergrad.

Other than the Christmas pageants the Baptist Sunday school put on every December and the musicals the senior class of Kernville High produced each spring, that *Henry* is the first theatrical performance John has ever seen. He is there mainly because Professor Gallagher has offered extra credit to anyone who attends, and John has done none too well on his *Faerie Queene* essay.

It seems strange to sit in a theater without a bag of popcorn and a coke, strange to be facing a stage instead of a screen. The audience is older than he'd expected, too, comprised of more professors and professionals from town than college students. While he waits for the play to begin, he tries to study the synopsis printed on his program, but the names mean nothing to him, and he finds the background information about Richard II and Bolingbrooke and Mortimer more confusing than edifying. He hopes he will not disgrace himself by clapping at the wrong place as he had earlier that fall when he'd taken a girl he'd thought he liked to hear a string quartet.

Then the curtains part, and suddenly the stage is filled with old men, the King of England—John gathers by the actor's crown and robe—and a retinue of lords and earls. Because he spent the previous summer memorizing *Romeo and Juliet,* the language is not all that hard to understand, but the politics they are discussing are both too brisk and too thick for him to follow. Stifling a sigh, he is settling in to wait for intermission when suddenly he hears the King expressing his disappointment in his son. *Yea, there thou mak'st me sad, and mak'st me sin*

> *In envy that my Lord Northumberland*
> *Should be the father to so blest a son—*
> *A son who is the theme of honor's tongue,*
> *Amongst a grove the very straightest plant,*

Whilst I, by looking on the praise of him,
See riot and dishonor stain the brow
Of my young Harry.

Listening to those lines John feels a pang. His own father has never been so openly critical of him, but he knows his dad's been disappointed by his lack of interest in sports and business. While John was home over Christmas, his father mentioned several times how Harve Rathmussen's boy was in the agricultural business program, how bright Jim's future looked. "It's an up and coming field," his dad suggested. "The scientific approach. What with the old-timers selling off their orchards, Harve says the big companies are hungry for bright young fellows to manage things for them."

John is still pondering his failures in his father's eyes when the scene changes, and instead of old men arguing politics, he is watching the king's disappointing son himself—the young Prince Hal—sparring and carousing with a loud, large-bellied rogue named Jack Falstaff.

In his English class the following week, when Professor Gallagher espouses the then-prevailing view that Falstaff is a coward and a dastard whose friendship Prince Hal must deny in order to become an honorable and upstanding king, John will feel as crimson-faced as Bardolph for having misread Jack Falstaff's character so completely, because that night in the theater, while he is discovering the story and meeting the characters for the first time, he falls in love with every aspect of that vast man—both the immortal Falstaff whose cry on the field of battle is *give me life*, as well as the immoral Jack who molds every moment to fit his own desires. By the time Professor Gallagher enumerates Dover Wilson's condemnations of the fat knight, it will be too late for John Wilson to renounce his love.

But he is smitten with Prince Hal that first night, too, having failed to detect Hal's cruelty toward Falstaff, or to notice any of the gibes that will later strike John as so obvious and unforgivable. Instead, he is seduced by the prince's languor, by his easy laughter and cool temper. In Hal's vow to redeem his misspent time when men least expect it, John thinks he recognizes a promise about himself.

Later, when he is introduced to the wasp-stung Hotspur, he also falls for him. Even though Hotspur is Prince Hal's rival, John thrills to hear him swear *it were an easy leap, To pluck bright honor from the pale-fac'd moon*, laughs when Hotspur claims he would keep the king's anger in motion by teaching a starling *to speak Nothing but 'Mortimer'*.

In subsequent scenes, John meets more of Falstaff's Boar's Head Tavern friends—crafty Poins, red-faced Bardolph, and Mistress Quickly, and he is introduced to more of the court folk, too—Hotspur's feisty wife and his feigning father, the superstitious Glendower, and Hal's valiant younger brother—and as each new scene unfolds, John longs to join the characters onstage, not as an actor—he has no desire to act, nor any illusions about his abilities in that arena—but as he, himself—John Hubbard Wilson—claiming his place among their bright revels and fierce battles.

Intermission arrives as an intrusion. He does not want to leave his seat, does not want to break the spell of the play for anything as inane as a cup of coffee or a visit to the can. Around him, he overhears conversations about cars and clothes and college politics, and he feels a hot indignation that anyone could discuss such mundane matters after what they have just observed. It reminds him of the angry pain he'd known at his mother's funeral when he spied Mr. Baker and Harve Rathmussen discretely shaking hands to firm up some business deal.

But when the house lights blink to signal the end of intermission, John feels an unexpected kinship with the people filing into the auditorium. As the theater rustles back to silence, he is suddenly struck by how they are all in that play together—he, the rest of the audience, the actors onstage—how the play is a thing they share, an act of communal imagining they are preparing to embark on.

Then he is lost again—or rather, once more captured and enraptured—his entire awareness cupped onstage. He has no idea what will happen next, no idea how the play will end. He hardly knows what to hope for. When King Henry tells his wayward son, *Thou hast redeem'd thy lost opinion*, John flushes with a vindication of his own. And when Falstaff is slain in battle at Shrewsbury, it does not matter to John that the villainous abominable misleader of youth once called his own soldiers warm slaves as he led them to their slaughter. Instead, tears burn John's sinuses as he watches Prince Hal kneel beside the vast corpse of his corpulent friend, lamenting that he could have better spared a better man. And when the prince trudges sorrowfully offstage, and the vast corpse leaps up and stabs dead Hotspur in the thigh, John gasps and laughs and does not care if he disgraces himself by clapping at that irreverent resurrection.

After the final round of politics that ends the play, after the audience's applause and the actors' curtain call, John gathers his jacket and program and heads out of the auditorium. Swept along with the other theatergoers, he is buoyed by a gratitude whose source he cannot quite locate, but which seems to extend beyond the play and its long-dead playwright, and even beyond the actors he has just seen leave the stage. In the lobby, the people chatting and flirting and fitting on their coats appear much more vivid and interesting than they had when he'd arrived. In their features and expressions he thinks he can catch glimpses of the people he has just met onstage.

"What did you think?" someone asks, and when no one else responds, John turns to find a coed looking directly at him as she slips her arms into her trench coat.

"Me?" he croaks, his voice stiff.

"Sure," she answers in defiance of the flush that is beginning to pink her neck beneath the sweep of her ponytail.

"I liked it."

"I saw you laughing."

"Actually, I liked it a lot." He feels strangely as if he has been caught at something, but glad, too, to have an opportunity to admit it.

"It's not true, you know," she suggests, coyly fitting a scarf over her head. As he watches her tie the ends beneath her chin, he is reminded of the pretty actress who played Mortimer's Welsh wife, the woman whose looks and kisses Mortimer could understand, although her language was a mystery to him.

"Not true?" he asks, pausing to hold the heavy door open for her and a small flood of other departing theatergoers, and then hurrying to catch up with her. "What do you mean?"

"The history isn't accurate. It compresses the time of Henry the Fourth's reign, and makes Prince Hal and Hotspur the same age when they were actually a generation apart." Stopping on the sidewalk beneath a streetlamp, she looks up at him speculatively. An iced wind twists between the trees. In the street-lit night, it is difficult to see if her blush persists.

He can hardly follow her criticisms, but even so, it troubles him to hear her finding fault with the play. It seems like looking for a flaw in the way a bird flies, like questioning a kiss, to criticize any aspect of what he has just witnessed.

"And of course there was no historical Jack Falstaff, either." She seems to be both teasing him and testing something, though he has no idea what, no idea how his answer might matter to her. Poised between annoyance and intrigue, he watches her, noticing the arch of her eyebrows, the curve of her lips, the way her scarf flutters in the dark breeze.

"So?" he says with a shrug and a grin.

"So you don't care about facts, about historical accuracy?"

"Damn facts and accuracy," he answers, offering her his arm with a gallantry that feels both novel and right. "It's truth I care about."

But here John wakes from his dream of that long-vanished time to find himself stranded in a worn leather chair, trapped in a wizened body and a strange, stiff, dizzy mind. A breeze wafting through the tree outside rouses the dappled shadows on the floor, and he wonders which truth that young swain thought he meant, Hotspur's ramrod attempt to shame the devil, Hal's plan to be better than his word, or Falstaff's bawdy claim that truth is like an old hostess—a man knows not where to have her.

It's truth I care about. The words ring faintly back to him as if from some performance he barely recalls attending. He wishes he knew more about the boy who spoke them—that ardent, awkward kid who shares his name. And he wishes he knew who she was, too—that bold, shy girl who dared to claim that Falstaff wasn't real. He wonders if she ever told him her name, wonders if she ever took his arm, wonders if they ever talked further about the play. But when he strains to follow those wonders any further, the images his mind finds shift like scarves in a cold wind—the scent of smoke, the taste of a kiss, a pair of empty glasses in a hotel bar—and before he can find the narrative that would explain what they might mean, the images drift away, leaving only a residue of loss where that story should have been.

"Tell me a story," an eager voice begs. It's a child's voice, lisp and pipe, and hearing it, John feels a wash of pleasure. *Tell me a story.* As he's claimed to many a class, humanity's craving for stories is more primal than the urge for sugar, perhaps more urgent than the ache for sex. It's stories that shape us, he likes to say, stories that give us purpose, stories that help us make sense of our strange lives.

"Merry or sad shall it be?" he asks the brown-eyed ghost-girl in his lap, and she twists around to study his face for a moment before she answers solemnly, "It's okay if no one gets married. But I don't like sad."

Chuckling with proprietary pleasure, he scoops up her hand, helps her to hold it steady while he pours Cracker Jack from the box into her palm. "How should I start?" he asks.

"You know," she answers, crunching contentedly.

"No, I don't," he teases.

"You know," she urges.

"Maybe I've forgotten."

"You haven't," she answers, complacently licking sugar from her fingers. "You wouldn't never forget."

"Give me a hint."

"It starts with one."

"One?" he echoes, momentarily genuinely perplexed.

"*Ssss*," she hisses. "One-*sssss* upon a time. And then you have to tell what there was. Once," she says again, tapping his leg as if he were a horse she was spurring forward. "Up. On. A. Time."

"Ahhh," he answers, savoring the sounds. "One—*sss* upon a time, there was . . ."

Then his memory seems to snag on another regret, though exactly what it is he cannot recall. Perhaps the story was too sad a tale, perhaps too full of sprites and goblins for the child's liking. Though instead of trying to solve that mystery and risk facing its final sting, John allows his thoughts to slip sideways instead.

Once upon a time, he ruminates—like the sad or fabulous old tales in *The Winter's Tale*. Or like *The Winter's Tale* itself, that fairy story of a play that flies on Time's swift wings from the wintery grim world of law-bound Sicilia to the lush, unruly shore of fair Bohemia. *Once upon a time*. He cannot now recall the name of the critic who first wrote about green worlds, but as sunlight crawls across the floor and inches up his legs to fill his empty lap with weightless gold, he remembers how once upon a time in a fit of midlecture inspiration, he'd found himself explaining the green world pattern in *The Winter's Tale* by comparing it to *The Wizard of Oz*, describing how alike Sicilia and stern, gray Kansas are, how much Bohemia resembles the wonderful world of Oz, and even how, when the characters return to Sicilia or Kansas in the final acts, they discover that what they have accomplished in their green worlds has transformed their homelands, too.

It's the victory of summer over winter, John rhapsodizes, the triumph of birth and growth over sere dead—

"Dad?" a voice asks, and John's brain echoes, *Dad*. But instead of lines and phrases, the associations that come to him are temperatures, weights, and textures, feelings beyond the hold of words. Ire and irritation, instant and hot. An old fury, long retained. And beneath that, a tug of love so strong it pulls the air from both his lungs.

"Dad?" the voice asks again. Twisting in his chair, John finds a woman standing at the threshold of his room. An eager, tentative woman with tousled hair and strangely familiar eyes, she waits at the doorway as if wanting to be invited in. She carries a book—a big, thick, gilt-edged thing that she clutches to her chest like a hopeful coed on her way to class.

He's seen her before, he's sure of that. He feels both wary and deeply pleased to see her now.

"Dad?" she says a third time, her voice tight and hopeful.

"Where have you been?" he answers at last, careful to keep his voice neutral.

"I visited back in April—remember?—not long after you moved in." She gives a swift wry shrug as she enters the room. "And here I am again." Her voice has that patina of professional cheer he has had to endure all too often of late. Lifting a hand from his lap, he gives a vague wave in her direction as if he were fending off a sorry sight. His hip is paining again today, his bones ache. He has spent the morning working—or attempting to, or wanting to—though it seems as if his efforts have all been stale and unprofitable, and he does not now remember accomplishing a thing.

"It's good to see you," the woman persists. "You're looking good." But when he shoots a glance at her, he can read the subtext in her eyes.

Still, he is tired enough of his own company that he beckons toward the empty chair he suddenly notices sitting like a small deus ex machina beside his own. "Sit," he urges. "Sit, sit. How are you? How've you been?"

Her expression freshens. She takes on a look of barely contained excitement that reminds John of the Christmasy anticipation of a child he'd once known. Lowering herself into the chair, she answers, "I've been fine, Dad, more than fine, actually. I just got some really great news—"

"Still in . . . coffee?" he asks.

"What?" The surprise on her face is replaced by a new swell of pleasure as she cries, "Yes, yes, I am!—I am still in coffee. You do know me!" she announces. "You remember me."

"'Whiles memory holds a seat in this distracted globe,'" he answers, tapping his forehead playfully. They share a smile that seems to curve between them like a rainbow. "Who's that?" John asks a second later, the smile still alive on his face.

"What?"

"Who says that? Who speaks that line?"

The grin on the woman's face does not waver even as she shakes her head. "I'm sorry, Dad. I'm afraid I don't know."

"Give it your best guess," he urges genially. "It's easy. He has more lines than any other . . . character."

"I really don't have a clue."

"You're not trying," he admonishes, but his voice is like a tickle, warm and teasing. In another moment he concedes, "It's Hamlet. The Great Dane," he adds to earn another of her smiles.

"Do you remember how you used to teach me lines?" she asks, her expression nearly wistful. "Back when you and Mom were still together?

I might have known it was Hamlet who said that about the distracted globe, but you left before we finished *Midsummer Night's Dream*."

"*I* left?" He gives her a sharp, stern look, shakes his head.

"You used to give me Cracker Jack when I got it right—'Lord, what fools these mortals be.' 'The course of true love never did run smooth.'"

An orange cat comes into view, creeping across the lawn as if stalking invisible prey. Like strangers on a bus, they watch as it places each paw daintily between the stems of grass, watch as it freezes for a moment in high attention, and then twists around to lick a hind leg.

"I've forgotten where you went to college," John tells the cat.

"I didn't, Dad," the woman answers. "I mean, I haven't yet, but— guess what?—yesterday I—"

"You never went to college?"

"It wasn't a good time, but now—"

"There was money, in the settlement. I made sure of that."

"Really? Well, maybe I can still use it," she says, her voice sparkling. "Because—get this—yesterday I got my acceptance letter—from the best school in the country! I can start in January. I haven't gotten my financial aid package yet," she prates, "so I don't know exactly how much it will cost me, but I know it's going to take a crazy lot of money, and I'm sure I can use all the help I—"

"Which best?" John breaks in to ask. "Harvard? Berkeley? There are any number that . . . aspire."

"Not Harvard or Berkeley," she answers gleefully. "Even better, for what I want to do. It's a college called ArtTech."

"I beg your pardon?"

"ArtTech."

"Impossible," he announces.

"According to *U.S. News*, it's the best school in the country for computer game development."

"Computer?"

"Computer game development." She speaks slowly, giving every syllable its due. "It's an entire college devoted to game research and development. It's ultracompetitive, especially for someone like me who's weak in math and programming. I still can't believe I'm in," she adds, shaking her head at the marvel of it all.

"Game . . . development?" In his mouth the words sound meager, or even vaguely obscene.

"It's a whole new field, Dad—interactive entertainment. It'll be an art someday, I'm sure of that. Right now, lots of games are still pretty much focused on sports or wars or errands, but what interests me is what else they can do, the world building and storytell—"

"Games."

"Not like games for kids—grownup stuff."

"Worse and worse."

"It fits with all the things I love," she pleads, "art and stories, imaginary worlds, people, and how they think. Remember how I used to make those lists back when I was a kid—people's names, with all kinds of facts about who they were and where they lived and what they did? Character profiles, you called them. I had whole notebooks full of them. And remember how I was always drawing pictures—people, landscapes, maps of made-up places? It's like now I can harness all of that. I'm not a good enough artist to do more than sketch concepts, but I do think I'll be good at helping to design quests and imagine worlds. It's hugely collaborative, and—"

"A girl . . . keen, as you."

"I thought you might at least be glad I'm going to college."

"I would be. If . . . you were." He knows a rise of pride at the aptness of his reply, but when he glances at the woman sitting next to him, he sees her visage sag as if she were aging before his eyes. He feels an unexpected twinge, though when he tries to think what he might do to slow her aging and ease his pang, he becomes so entwisted in a complicated narrative of motives, plots, and damages that he has to let the whole thing drop.

They sit in silence, like strangers waiting for the next stop.

"I've been thinking, about green worlds," he offers eventually.

"Oh." Her tone is empty.

"In the plays."

"Of course."

He shoots her a sharp look, but his voice is mild when he says, "Like *The Wizard of Oz*. Only, richer, of course, denser, more . . . true. In the comedies, and in the romances, too, how the characters leave their normal worlds, their courts or . . . cities . . . behind, and then come transmuted—transformed, I mean. As illogical, and in . . . evitable, as the change from caterpillar to . . . butterfly. It's a question of what triggers all that . . . change, or enables it, perhaps. I was thinking about art, but there's also, nature. Though always it seems, it takes . . . a tragedy, some split, or vast . . . calamity. Regeneration, too, and seasonal."

He sighs. Giving her a wry grimace as if to apologize for his inability to capture his thought and bring it back alive, he says, "The Green Man was a trickster. Don't, forget."

"Okay," she answers cautiously, her voice nearly curving the word into a question.

"Here, look, Dad," she adds, suddenly thrusting the brick of the book she has been hugging in his direction, "I brought you a present."

It is a gaudy thing, he sees when she sets it in his lap, bound in maroon leatherette, embossed with gilt lettering. A copy of the Chandos portrait—what they used to call the sexy Shakespeare—decorates its cover. John studies the sitter's features, the wise and wary eyes, the balding forehead, tidy beard and jaunty earring, the sensitive, sensual lips—lips for speaking, lips for kissing—lips that seem nearly ready to indulge their own Mona Lisa smile.

"Well, well," John murmurs, feeling once more that wistful tug, his wish to know the man who may have owned that face nearly erotic in its pull. "Will."

"William Shakespeare," the woman offers eagerly, pointing to the golden words, "See, it says here—*Complete Works.*"

"Complete," John echoes, scrutinizing those inscrutable eyes and reflecting that it has always been no more possible to name their expression than it has been to pin down Shakespeare's own opinions in his plays.

When he makes no effort to open the book, Miranda retrieves it from his lap. Opening it herself, she pages to the table of contents. "What was your favorite play, Dad?" she asks, scanning attentively down the list. "What *is* your favorite, I mean."

"Favorite?" After a long moment he adds, "Someone said picking . . . one play." He gives a slow sad sigh, "Is like choosing a favorite, child." A frown passes across his brow, followed by the tremble of a smile. "But I only ever had . . . the one."

"Which one?" she prompts, and seems to hold her breath.

He is quiet for a long while more, looking out the window to where roses blow in the summer air, where soldiers are gathering for battle, and young women are dressed as boys, where tempests are brewing, and lovers are swearing their fervent vows.

"*Love's Labor's Won,*" he announces at last, with a finality that makes it seem that something of great import has just at that moment been settled.

"*Love's Labor's Won?*" Miranda echoes. "Oh. Your favorite play." Running her finger dutifully down the table of contents, she adds, "Funny—I don't see that one here. Here's *Love's Labor's Lost,*" she offers, "in the comedies. Do you mean *Love's Labor's Lost?*"

"No." He shakes his head. "*Won.*"

"*Love's Labor's Won?* Are you sure?" She bends back over the book. "I don't see *Won* here anywhere."

He gazes into the garden for so long it seems he's vanished into whatever's left inside his head while she closes the book gently and sets it on the dresser. A small while later, he speaks again. "It's lost."

"What's lost?" she asks, "You mean, your favorite play's *Love's Labor's Lost*?"

"No, *Won*—*Love's Labor's Won* is lost. It was registered. But no copies . . . appear. It's lost," he repeats. "Gone, and . . . forgotten. Dead and," he sighs, "rotten."

"Oh. Well, wow. So *Love's Labor's Won* was lost, but it's your favorite play?" she asks, leaning towards him as if her question might help keep him in the room with her.

"Yes."

"But why, Dad?" After a quiet moment she offers, "Because love won?"

"Because," he says impatiently, "it could be anything. It's what we don't . . . have, what we can only imagine. The . . . possibilities.

"But you look good," he says, returning from his musings to look at her directly. "I like your . . ." his hand circles on his wrist as though he could conjure the word from midair. "Excrements," he offers at last. "Your shorn locks," he explains, gesturing toward her hair.

"My hair?" she gives a nervous laugh, lifts her hand to brush the crown of her head. "Oh, well. Thanks. I—"

"Purple is a noble color," he announces. "But not for hair." After a moment he adds, "It's good to see you."

"It's good to see you, too, Dad," she answers swiftly, "I'm—"

"It was good of you, to come."

Emotions flicker across her face like the shadows of racing clouds.

"Dad?" she says at last. Her voice is nearly shrill. "Last time you asked me what I wanted, why I was here. And I said that I only wanted to see you. But maybe that wasn't entirely true."

"Nothing ever is," he tells the cat who sits sphinxlike in the sun.

"I wanted to see you again, of course. But also, I wanted to talk, to . . . try to get things straight."

"Straight," he speculates, testing the word, sounding it, weighing meanings, inviting associations.

"I didn't want to leave things like—the way they've been between us. I wanted—I mean I'd like to—"

"To come to terms," he offers.

"Exactly!" she announces. "To come to terms."

"Okay," he agrees. Looking fully into her face, he adds, "all right."

For a moment their eyes seem to hold an entire world between them. Then, giving her a friendly nod, John returns his attention to the cat who has begun to clean its nether end, one leg lifted off the ground with the precision of a dancer.

Leaning toward him, Miranda waits, but when he fails to add anything more, she finally opens the silence to suggest, "I'd like to talk about what happened in London—to tell you what really happened, I mean, to me."

At the sound of her voice suddenly so tight with pain, an ache seizes John's chest like the cramps he used to feel as a kid when he'd run too far too fast. He studies the cat carefully, in hopes of not upsetting the precious concord he and she have so lately agreed upon.

"I know I said some pretty strong things to you," she persists, "and I'm sorry about that. But I think you might understand more if you knew what happened from my point of view."

He has no idea what she is talking about, but her devastated expression puts him in mind of *Troilus and Cressida*. "'Understand more clear,'" he intones dolefully, "'What's past and what's to come is strew'd with husks And formless ruin of oblivion.'"

It's a grim, sad line, he knows, and, in an attempt to cheer them both, he asks, "Who's that? What play?"

"I don't know, Dad," she sighs. "I thought we were talking about us."

"We are," he quips. "We're talking as we . . . speak."

"But can't you please just talk plain English, instead of quoting Shakespeare all the time?" Her voice sharpening, she pleads, "For once, can't you please just speak for yourself?"

"Shakespeare," he says with quiet dignity, "speaks for all of us."

She takes a quick, sharp breath. But in the next instant she seems to catch herself. Exhaling as carefully as if she were trying to keep a candle flame alight, she suggests, "But what I want to know has to do with you and I, not Shakespeare," she suggests.

"You and me," he offers not unkindly. "You want the . . . objective case."

"Oh, Dad—" she gasps.

"Should we go?" he interjects.

"Well, not right—"

"We don't have much time," he frets, twisting in his seat to glance at the open door.

"I'm sorry, Dad," she answers wanly. "I'm afraid I just don't know."

"You're sorry?" he barks, instantly incensed. Turning to look her full in the face, he thunders, "You just don't know? Here I've been waiting all this time, waiting for you to come—waiting and waiting and waiting—and now that you're here, you just don't . . . know?" Waving off her remonstrations, he hisses, "It's too late now. It's over. Dead and, rotten. You ruined everything."

Outside, Randi stands on the white sidewalk, still stunned by the weight of the July heat that met her the instant she burst through the building's heavy front doors, and stunned, too, by the size of her disappointment, by her foolishness for being there at all. She'd known better than to risk another visit. She'd reasoned her way back through the whole sorry story so many times, and every time she'd come to the same stark conclusion. The man who was her father was already gone—both the daddy who'd teased her and taught her lines from Shakespeare, and the father who'd excised her from his life for being such a messed-up teenager. When she'd tried to visit the husk that remained, it had only agitated what little was still left of him. He was right about that, at least, she thinks with a bitter smirk—it's too late now.

That first visit had been hard on her, too, harder than she'd expected, rousing longings she'd hardly known she still harbored, conjuring shames she'd thought she'd put to rest, filling her dreams with images that troubled her for days—bleeding books and leering boys and sharp-toothed rodents with weeping human eyes. She'd decided back in April that nothing would be gained by visiting him again, that little would be lost if she never returned.

It made no sense to add to his confusion and her disappointment by forcing him to endure another meeting. Even if it did occur to him, in some brief lucid moment, that although he'd once had a daughter, his daughter never visited him anymore, she doubted he would care all that much. And if he did sometimes feel a pang—if he missed her for a moment or even yearned for her for a day or so—wasn't that a kind of justice? When she was ten and twelve and sixteen and even eighteen, the ache of his absence had been as constant as an ulcer, as impossible to ignore as a grain of sand in her eye. If he missed her occasionally now, wasn't that only fair?

"More than fair," Mink had agreed back in early June when she was still trying to justify her decision. It had been the evening of another unseasonably hot day, and they were sitting in the kitchen, courting any wisp of breeze that might waft through the open windows. She'd been home from work only long enough to open a Coke and trade her coffee-scented uniform for a tank top and a pair of running shorts. Mink was working on a chart of types of stars for his summer science class, while she sat facing the window, idly rolling the icy can across her neck and chest and staring at the tangle of black wires, leaves, and branches that blocked her full view of the darkening sky.

"It's called logical consequences, Ran," Mink said, glancing up from his work. "Especially since your dad was the supposed grown-up when things went south, I'd say your biggest responsibility now is to protect yourself."

It was what she had been telling herself all along, but coming from Mink, it suddenly sounded wrong. Setting her lips to the opening of her can, she took a slug, welcoming the tangy sweetness, the carbonation widening in her throat. She sighed, "It's just that I keep having this superstitious feeling like I'll be missing out on something important if I don't go back. Though frankly," she added with a dark laugh, "I'm not sure I'd know what was important even if I was there to see it."

"Whaddya mean?" An open bag of corn chips sat on the table between them. Setting down his marker, Mink rustled in the bag for a handful.

"He went in and out of focus so fast. How could I ever know for sure what was him talking and what was his—" Randi held out an empty hand, "—condition? I swear there were moments when he was all there, when we seemed so close to really being connected. But the next minute he wasn't making any sense at all. Not like he was in a fog, but like he *was* a fog." She took a swallow from her Coke, "Like my father was nothing but fog."

"Actually, he's not fog, he's bacteria."

"Huh?"

"We all are. Our bodies are twenty times more bacteria than cells. It's true." He grinned at her grimace. "My class went ape when I told them that. Twelve-year-olds love that kind of shit."

"Stuff," she offered, shaking her head at the wackiness. "You'll have to learn to clean up your language if you want to keep that job." She pulled a chip from the bag, but as she lifted it toward her mouth, it suddenly looked so stiff and flat it was hard to recognize it as food. She set it on the table instead. "I keep thinking he just needs defragging." She crushed the chip against the table with the palm of her hand.

"Ran," Mink said quietly. Reaching across his work, he placed a fingertip at the corner of her eye, and then, tenderly, he traced the path a tear might take down her cheek. "People can't be defragged." He let his hand fall from her face to cover hers where it lay empty on the table.

"I know," she said flatly. "It's game over. My dad's already gone. For better and worse, no one gets to respawn."

"Fathers come in a lot of flavors," he added gently. Picking up her hand, he pressed its knuckles to his lips, and then, returning her hand to her, he swept the chip crumbs off the table and popped them into his mouth. "Sometimes you just get a dud," he said nearly cheerfully. "A dud dad—like mine."

"I know about dud parents. Look at my mom, for fuck's sake. But with my dad," she sighed. "I'm not so sure. For a long time I actually believed we would have another chance someday, that somehow there would still be time." Outside the open window, she saw a tiny shine amid the tangle of wires and branches, the night's first star. She wondered how old that light was, light from some deep past, light that would travel on and on, long after the star itself was gone. She said, "Stupid me. All that ever did was keep the pain alive."

Gently Mink said, "What happened in London was not your fault."

Despite the tenderness of his tone, his words reached her before she was prepared to hear them. She winced, then shook her head so fiercely it was as if she were trying to shake tears back inside her eyes. "My dad used to say if you're any good at all, it's your own damn fault."

"I think Hemingway said that first," Mink replied wryly.

"Not Shakespeare?" she answered with a grateful smirk. "Anyway, I would rather be my own damn fault than someone else's victim. You would, too, if you'd grown up with my mom."

"So there we are," he'd answered gently, taking up another marker and returning to his poster, "back to my point exactly. The best way to keep from being a victim is to write your own terms."

It sounded right at the time. That evening, as other stars assumed their places in the sky and the day's heat dissolved into the balmy night, it had made sense to cut old losses, made sense to protect the new self she was laboring to become. It seemed right to let her father go, for good and all.

But last week the landline rang as she was leaving for work, and she'd scooped up the phone to find Sally on the other end, saying, "I've been thinking it would be good for John if you and I staggered our visits." Randi stood at the kitchen counter in her black slacks and clean shirt, staring at the peels and shells and grounds in the overflowing compost bucket, as Sally went on: "I'd be happy to work around your schedule."

"I'm not going back," Randi blurted, suddenly regretting that she hadn't called Sally to tell her that, ruing her sense that she now owed Sally something.

"Not going back?"

"I don't think my visit did him any good. He was pretty upset by the time I left."

"Really?" Sally's puzzlement sounded genuine. "The shift nurse said John seemed much happier after you left, and when I asked him about it later, he told me he was glad you'd come, that he wanted to see you again."

He'd driven down to Santa Cruz to see her, not long after he and Freya returned from Spain, when the fallout from her misadventure in London was still spreading like a silent poison through her entire self and soul, even as she strained to pretend that what happened had really been no big deal.

She'd given her mother the same streamlined version of events that she'd outlined for her dad, only, unlike him, Barb had been entirely sympathetic with Randi's point of view. It wasn't Randi's fault she'd gotten lost, Barb said indignantly. It wasn't Randi's fault that her dad's little Shakespeare thing just happened to be the next day, and it certainly wasn't Randi's fault that John always believed that whatever he did was so much more important than what anyone else was doing. Her father was a pig, Barb announced. She'd been saying so for years, and now that Randi was older, she could see it for herself. Her father should be sued or shot or put in jail for sending Randi home when her only mistake was getting lost and staying out a little too long.

Randi herself had still not been able to fit what she could recall of that night into a story that would explain what truly happened, though in reality she had not tried very hard. On her flight back to California, she'd managed to reduce the entire episode to a bitter joke, telling herself she was lucky to have found a way to skip that bogus trip to Spain, telling herself it was okay if she couldn't remember everything, since as soon as she put it out of her mind entirely, it would be as if it had never happened at all.

To pass the time while she waited to forget, she started fooling around on the computer her father had handed down to her the previous spring in hopes it would help improve her schoolwork. She began by playing the solitaire game the computer came with, and then she resurrected *The Oregon Trail* game she'd played as a kid. But after a few weeks she graduated to *Doom*.

She got the game from a boy she'd secretly liked for years, one on the fringes of the crowd she hung around. Before London she would have been more thrilled by his attention than curious about the video game he offered to share with her. But when they ran into each other at the park where her group liked to congregate on balmy evenings, and he handed her the yellow floppy disk that contained the first episode of *Doom*, suggesting that if she liked it, maybe they could get together sometime and play through to the end, wariness prickled through her like a thousand electric shocks. She'd made up an excuse to leave the park right away, and for months she didn't go back again.

Barb was already out by the time Randi got home, so she was spared having to explain herself or spend the evening comforting her mother. Grabbing a Coke, a banana, and a bag of chips, and trading her black velvet skirt and Doc Martens for a tee shirt and sweats, she booted up her computer, pushed the yellow disk into the drive, and watched with a kind of listless impatience while the game loaded and the letters that spelled out *DOOM* rose up to dominate the screen. Suddenly, she was inside a strange dark building, urgent electronic music was playing, and at the bottom of the screen a masculine hand that seemed to belong to her was pointing a pistol at the roaring red monsters lunging in her direction.

She died in that first instant, and afterwards she died about a million times more. But click by click she figured out how to manipulate the mouse so she could move smoothly down the strange dark corridors of the Phobos hangar, click by click learned how to keep her health up, collect weapons, avoid green slime, and kill more and more of the steady stream of shotgun guys and zombies that wanted to attack her.

She liked that she had to concentrate so entirely on something that seemed like life or death in the moment but that had no meaning beyond the glowing screen. She liked that she could see her skills improving, slowly but measurably. She enjoyed the sizzle of adrenaline she felt when she was attacked, and she took a pleasure almost deeper than she was comfortable with in the groans and roars of the invaders when her shots hit them, in the satisfying red splats they made when they died. It was gratifying to go back through parts of the hangar she had already traversed and see the bloodied corpses of those she'd slain still scattered across the tesselated floors. And even back then, in that stilted, gruesome first-person shooter, she'd been fascinated by the entire world the game suggested, the glimpses it gave her of dark corners and strange mountains and unexplored distant vistas.

When the doorbell rang on Sunday afternoon, she was still wearing the sweats she'd put on the night before. With a couple of breaks for naps and snacks and to pacify her mother, she'd been playing steadily ever since, working as hard as she'd ever worked on anything. After hours of butt-numbing focus and tooth-gnashing frustration, she had finally picked up her first shotgun and was beginning her forays into the nuclear plant, so that at first she had no intention of answering the door. But when the bell sounded for the third time, she assumed that Barb had locked herself out again. Pausing her game reluctantly, and rising a little dizzily, she'd stumbled to the door.

"Dad," she gasped when she saw him standing there. He was wearing his weekend jeans and sports jacket, and an expression that seemed both penitent and stern. "Hi," she added lamely while waves of shame and pain the size of the monsters at Mavericks Beach broke over her.

"Didn't your mother tell you I was coming?" he asked, eying her disheveled clothes, her rumpled hair, and unwashed face.

"She must of forgot."

"Must have forgotten," he suggested mildly.

"Whatever."

"Where is she?" he asked as she stepped back to let him pass through the door, and then watched as he took in the meager squalor of their living room, the threadbare sofa and the nearly new TV.

"At work?" she said with a shrug, hoping it wouldn't occur to him that the office her mother managed was closed on Sundays.

"So," he said, infusing his voice with so much false cheer that Randi was almost embarrassed for him. "What've you been up to today?"

"Playing a game," she admitted, wincing at her sudden awareness of how that would only underscore all her previous failures in her father's eyes.

"A game?" he asked. "By yourself? What kind of game?"

"A computer game," she answered.

"A *computer* game?"

She shrugged. "It's better than watching crappy TV or taking drugs."

"Are drugs and TV your only alternatives?"

"Maybe," she answered, her tone a mix of desperation and defiance.

"I'd like to think your world could be a richer place than that. I know it could, if you wanted it to."

"Whatever."

"How've you been?"

"Okay." She found an unexpected pleasure in watching him struggle to overcome the annoyance their conversation was causing him.

"School off to a good start?" he asked with more fake heartiness.

"I guess." Without warning, she found herself back inside that moment in London when the policemen who returned her to the hotel finally left, and she was alone in the room with her father. She'd been dirty and sore and scared and beyond exhausted, but the relief of being back with him flooded her like warm syrup. For a second she felt so overjoyed that she would have started giggling if the sight of his face— as cold and set and stern as stone—hadn't shocked her out of it.

"What classes are you taking this fall?" he asked now, frowning at the TV screen.

"The usual crap—English," she began, and then, before he could react, she added, "and math and history and stuff."

He sighed. "Miranda, I really wish you'd talk with me."

"I am talking," she quipped. "I'm talking right now."

"I want you to know that I feel as bad about what happened on our trip as I'm sure you do."

Terror surged through her—terror and shame and oceans of regret—while he continued, "I hated to have to send you home. But really, I had no choice. When you're older, you'll understand."

But it seemed she understood right then. Suddenly, all her sorry, muddled feelings crystallized into a single emotion—an anger so sharp and clear it seemed capable of cutting granite. She saw what she had never seen before, that her father was the problem, the reason she'd felt so dirty and stupid and forlorn. Suddenly she hated him, and not just for sending her home from London in disgrace, but for being so judgmental, so unwilling to value anything about her but the things he thought he already understood.

He said, "It's obvious that we both have some work to do to rebuild our relationship. But I think it will be worth it. I know we still have a lot to give each other."

"What relationship?" she asked coldly, and it was like blasting another zombie with her newly acquired shotgun to watch the concern drain from his face.

"Fuck you, Dad," she'd said, riding her elation. "Just totally fuck you."

After he left and she'd rammed the door shut behind him, she returned to the starting alcove of the nuclear plant exhilarated by both her clarity and her courage, convinced that she could become the person she wanted to be, now that she was free of her father.

But she never felt that free again, and as she trudged on through the weeks of that grim fall, she began to suspect that whatever actually happened in London, she would never be able to leave that night behind. When her nausea increased and her suspicions grew, she lost interest in chainsawing monsters and finding her way to Hell. She returned to her childhood *Oregon Trail*, taking a kind of mindless comfort in naming the members of her travel party, choosing her supplies at Matt's general store, and then starting off on what the old-fashioned type font in the dialogue box promised would be a long and difficult journey. When a member of her party died of typhoid or diphtheria, she felt as much relief as failure, glad to be rid of even the imaginary burden of someone else's life.

Every night when she went to bed, she lay under the rumpled

covers grinding through her real-life dreads, trying not to imagine the long and difficult journey that was in store for her no matter what choices she made, managing to sleep only when she had promised herself yet again that she would do something about it in the morning.

Finally, when she still hadn't had a period by the end of October, she went to a pharmacy on the other side of town where she spent a week's lunch money on a home pregnancy test. The next morning, she dipped the plastic wand in the vial with her pee, and when the second blue line appeared beside the one the instructions called the control, there was a long moment before she could comprehend what it meant. Standing in the cluttered bathroom, with her mother yelling through the locked door that she couldn't find her car keys, shoes, and aspirin, she'd felt a gut punch of pure despair.

Dad, her heart cried silently before she could think to stop it. *Daddy, I need you.*

Burying the wand at the bottom of the full wastebasket, she'd left the bathroom to help her mother find her things and get to work. Then, pleading an imaginary period, she stayed home from school, vacillating between sick panic and a state of numb despondence as she tried to decide what her next step should be.

It seemed certain that whatever she ended up doing, at some point she would need the help—or at least the money—of an adult. At first she thought it would be impossible to reach out to her father. But he was smarter, calmer, less hysterical than her mother. She couldn't help hoping that if he only knew the truth, he would feel at least some bit of obligation toward her. Besides, Barb had been drinking a lot that fall, and Randi worried that if anything happened to make her drink still more, she might lose her job, and they would end up on the streets or camping down at the levee.

When she calculated that it was late enough for her dad to be home from work but still too early for her mom to walk in on their conversation, she went into the kitchen where the phone was stationed and dialed her father's number. Clutching the receiver like a life raft, she listened as it rang and rang and rang.

She had just convinced herself that no one was home, when someone finally answered. At the sound of Freya's smug hello, Randi's first impulse was to hang up, but in the split second in which she had to make that decision, she reminded herself it might be days before she could find another time to try to reach her father without her mother knowing about it.

"It's Randi," she'd said, struggling to crush the quaver in her voice. "Is my dad there?"

"No," Freya answered. And then waited.

"I want to talk to him. Do you know when he'll be back?"

"Not sure."

"Well, maybe . . . do you think you could maybe have him call me?"

"I'll *tell* him you called," Freya answered with icy precision. "But it's not my place to *have* him do anything for you. He'll have to make those decisions for him—"

To keep from sobbing into the receiver, Randi hung up before Freya could finish. Then, stumbling back through the silent apartment, she'd thrown herself on her bed, given herself up to crying while she waited for her father to call her back.

But by the time Barb staggered in at ten, Randi had run out of tears and her father still hadn't called. He didn't call the next day, or the next day, or the next. He never called at all until her birthday, and by then it hardly mattered, since three days after she'd tried to reach him, she'd been seized by the wickedest period she'd ever known, with hours of cramps that stabbed like knives and floods of blood and, in the end, a little wad of tissue like a crushed raspberry that Randi guessed was meant to be a baby.

"You still there?" she heard Sally ask inside her ear. Pushing back against those memories, Randi answered, "He got mad when I said I'd never gone to college, and even madder when I wouldn't help him leave. In the end, I'd say he seemed pretty darn clear about not wanting me there."

"Oh, no," Sally answered ardently. "That's just not true. One of the first things your father ever told me about you was how much he wanted to be back in touch."

When those words registered inside her head, Randi closed her eyes as if the little darkness she found there might somehow protect her from their power. But alone in the blackness behind her eyelids, she'd felt more vulnerable instead of less. A memory popped into her head, entire and unbidden, how one Easter when she was six or eight, the Easter Bunny had left a bright little envelope in her basket along with the usual jelly beans and chocolate eggs. *Instant Life!* it claimed on the front of the package, and when she'd emptied the teaspoon of dusty powder it contained into a glass of water, she'd watched, transfixed, as tiny translucent creatures appeared, frolicking in what moments earlier had been only water, drifting and dancing like minute living feathers—revived, her daddy had explained, from microscopic cysts which could remain dormant for many years. Hope was like that, she'd thought angrily—translucent, ephemeral, and resurrected from the most unlikely dust.

When she opened her eyes, the compost bucket was still there, still heaped with sour scraps, and Sally was saying, "I know there's more than one side to any story, and more than one way to interpret every side. But I also know your father's missed you. He loves you. And now he's old. And sick. And you're his only child.

"He's not going to get any better," Sally continued before Randi could find a way to answer, "but he does have better days. I'm sure it was a surprise for him, to see you again after all those years. It probably confused him, maybe stirred up memories or feelings he hasn't been aware of for a while. Maybe he was tired, or maybe his hip was acting up. It's not a good idea to get it replaced now, and sometimes he's in a lot of pain.

"I know it's not my place to ask it," she added after a pause, "but I really wish you'd give him another chance."

And so she'd let herself get duped once more. Though now, standing on the hot sidewalk with her father's final words still clanging in her head, Randi promises herself it won't happen again. What's done is done, she thinks grimly, groping in her bag for a cigarette and her lighter as she follows the sidewalk around the building to the little smoking outpost in the back.

It was also dumb to buy that book for him, she tells herself as she pries a cigarette from her pack and lights it. When she'd seen that copy of *The Complete Works* in the window of the bookstore next to the coffee shop, she'd thought of her dad immediately, imagined how his face would light up at the sight of it. She'd hoped that having it might help to fill his empty days, and even that his pleasure might somehow help to reconcile the two of them. *Reconcile*, she thinks drily—like making the contents of the register at work jive with the day's transactions. After a busy shift, it can sometimes take forever to find those last odd pennies. Occasionally, she cheats, adding a little money of her own to the till. To pay for her stupidity, is how she thinks of it.

With a fresh sweep of chagrin, she recalls her father's book-filled office at the university, the walls of books he'd always had at home. If owning a copy of Shakespeare's plays was still important to him, surely his new wife would have seen that he had one.

Staring at the smoke unfurling from her cigarette, Randi recalls their confusion about her father's favorite play: *It's won . . . it's lost . . . Love's Labor's Won is lost.* It was like some kind of comedy of errors, she thinks, like that old Abbott and Costello baseball skit Mink showed her on YouTube—*Who's on first, What's on second, I Don't Know's on third.*

Once, her father would have enjoyed that joke himself. He'd had a sense of humor, back when she'd thought she'd known him best. It could be subtle, to be sure—sometimes too dry for a little girl to understand, though at other times he could be flat-out silly. She remembers him observing, "Well roared, Lion," when she farted at the dinner table, how even her mother's scowl had not prevented him from adding something about her rank offense smelling to heaven. She remembers giggling so hysterically that she'd inadvertently roared again, loudly enough that even her mother had joined their laughter in the end.

She sits for a moment, enervated and inert. But suddenly, the thought of her ArtTech acceptance comes welling up, irrepressible as the corny helium balloon Mink bought to congratulate her with, effervescent as the bubbles in the champagne he'd poured. Yesterday morning when she'd first opened the email, she'd read the message over and over, confused by that word, "Congratulations!," convinced it must have some alternate meaning that she was too dumb to understand, afraid to believe the simple truth that she had been accepted at ArtTech, that she was in. Now, despite her father's rejection, despite the heat and the sour-sweet smells wafting from the dumpsters at the far end of the building, she finds herself buoyant with pride and anticipation once again.

She wishes she could have got him to appreciate even the smallest inkling of what that degree will mean to her, how thrilled she is to have a chance to play at least a little part in developing an art the world has not yet known.

Recently, she's realized she has another ambition, too, one that's been growing parallel to her first desire. Because in addition to helping to shape a new way to enthrall, move, soothe, and challenge an audience, she hopes to expand the roles for girls and women in computer games. She'd thought things would have evolved already, as more and more girls became gamers. But most of the new games are still as unenlightened as ever. Most of the protagonists are still straight males—and most of the playable characters are, too—while all too many of the women are still only props, prizes, or plot devices.

She's tired of playing characters in chain-mail bikinis, tired of playing games where getting the girl is the end goal and playing like a girl is the ultimate insult. She wants to make games where women rescue themselves. Lately, she keeps thinking of the kid she'd been in London—that eager, gullible girl who was so unable to say or do what she needed to in order to change the outcome of that evening. She can't escape the feeling that some part of her is still pinned on that fetid bed in that sordid room. And she also can't shake her faith that she will somehow be helping to free that mute, caught girl—if only she can create the games she dreams of making.

She is already bracing herself to find out exactly what her education will cost. Her letter from ArtTech said financial aid information would be forthcoming, and now that she knows she has been accepted, she plans to start looking for scholarships right away. For months Mink has been promising her they will find a way to pay, and she has been telling herself that if she can only get in, she won't let herself be defeated by anything as dumb as money. For a moment, when her father mentioned that education fund, she'd thought she'd stumbled across the perfect cheat, a way to please her father at the same time that it eased the way for her.

But as the smoke from her cigarette spills upward into the hot still air, she concedes it was actually lucky that her visit turned out as badly as it had, since however much or little that fund might have contained, it would have been disastrous for her to accept even a dime of it. It was money he'd set aside back when she was still his princess, she thinks sourly, money he'd no doubt believed would pay off any debts he might owe her and at the same time buy himself the kind of daughter he would be proud of having—a daughter with degrees from

Harvard or Berkeley—like experience points he could earn to level up in some stupid game.

"So this guy goes to the doctor," a voice behind her announces, and she twists around to see the man she met last time—Toby? Tony?—walking toward her, his cigarette already emptying smoke into the hot air. "And he's naked, except for a layer of plastic wrap."

Dropping into the chair next to hers, he continues, "'Doc,' the guy goes, 'what's wrong with me?' 'I don't know,' his doctor answers, 'but I can clearly see your nuts.'"

Before she can decide whether to wince or laugh, he holds his hands up as if to prove he's carrying no weapons. "Okay, okay. Then how about this one: What did the elephant ask the naked man?"

"What?" she asks with a helpless shake of her head.

"How do you eat with that little thing?"

"Groan," she says.

"How's your dad?" he asks, grinning.

"Who knows?" she answers brusquely.

"That bad?"

"He said I ruined everything." She tries to make her voice light, to offer that fact like her own black joke, but the sudden wobble in her chest prevents her. Stinging with chagrin, she stares at the wall where the ivy dangles in the heat like limp misshapen hearts.

"He didn't mean it," he says.

"And you know this because?"

"You wouldn't be here if he did. Besides." For a moment he is quiet, as if he were dipping back into his own thoughts. "I think a lot of what the residents say is like the stuff you'd say in dreams—not what you really mean, or even what you might think but wouldn't actually say, but just whatever happens to bubble up when the pot gets stirred." He waves his hand, and the smoke from his cigarette describes a complicated curlicue in the hot air. "Foam, or something. Froth. You can't take the bad stuff personally."

"But if I can't take the bad stuff personally, doesn't that mean I can't take the good stuff personally, either?"

"Oh, no." He grins. "The good stuff he means."

She shudders. "If I ever get like that, I just hope I can remember how to pull the trigger."

He tastes his cigarette thoughtfully, studies her through the smoke. "You say that now. But most of the residents, they seem happy enough. About as happy as the rest of us, I'd say. They go through phases, of course. And sundowners can be a pain. But maybe even sundowning isn't really all that bad. I mean, they don't seem bothered by it later. Alive's alive, after all. It beats the alternative, at least if you're not in a pile of pain."

"He can't think. He can hardly remember a thing," Randi answers bitterly. She is afraid to question him about phases or ask what sundowning means.

"Maybe it's not all that important," her smoking partner offers, "thinking, remembering. He can still see the sun and smell the flowers. He can still enjoy my cooking. Heck, *he* can probably still laugh at my jokes—which is more than I can say about some people," he adds pointedly.

"I would just want to be dead," she says.

"Does your dad want to be dead?"

"I don't know. He doesn't know," she adds disgustedly. "But I'll tell you one thing, the man he used to be would want to be dead."

"People change. Maybe he's not that man anymore."

"What are you, some kind of damn philosopher?"

"Me?" Spewing smoke, he gives a blunt laugh. "I'm a cook. He didn't mean it," he adds gently, "about you ruining everything."

Water fills her eyes as instantly as if he had just flung ash-filled sand into her face. Giving a vague wave, she stumbles away down the sidewalk. She realizes she needs to be driving. Suddenly, she is desperate to be racing along the freeway—anonymous and alone— with the windows open so the wind can whip the tears from her cheeks and ruffle her hair like a rough hand. She craves the punch and scrape of music, too, something metal, something feral. And mindless, she thinks with a shudder as the irony of it hits her. She wants music and motion to wipe away her mind.

Something has gone wrong.

Some deeply troublous thing has happened, though John can't at this moment identify just what. Instead, he paces the room like a caged lion, circling the floor with a gait both impatient and abstracted as he tries to hammer out exactly what is plaguing him. He wants to work his way through his confusion, wants to discern what has been suffered, to understand where blame lies and what the remedy might be.

In the comedies, confusion leads to understanding. In the tragedies, it's suffering that does. In the romances, it's a strange blend of both. But now when John tries to understand his confusion or to name what he has suffered, he is overcome with the same dull-headed dizziness he's felt of late when he attempts to study his investment statements or peer beneath the hood of Sally's car. Like poor honest Cassio after that monster Iago has got him drunk, John remembers a mass of things, but none distinctly.

Distractedly, he circles the room, stalking the epiphany that seems to orbit just out of reach, the explanation for why he feels so hurt and irked, the reason everything seems grim and doomed. "Think," he snarls to himself, gnashing his teeth and growling with frustration.

"Think," he commands, banging his forehead with his fist, hitting so hard he feels the hurt of it in both his knuckles and his temples. "Think, for Christsake, think."

But in that moment it seems he has forgotten how.

He falls into his chair, clutching the arms, squeezing until his nails carve crescents into the worn leather, until his own arms tremble with the effort. "Think," he growls, bashing the chair's arm with the full weight of his fist. It's what he's so often urged his students when they seek him out with questions about the essays they are writing. "Think," he'll say, his tone encouraging or commanding, depending on their individual personalities and how hard he's seen them work. *What exactly are you arguing here? How else might you support that claim? What other examples can you find? How could you account for this fact, too? How might these insights be connected?*

But, although he strains until his temples throb, he cannot identify the argument, cannot locate the main idea, cannot even remember exactly what it is he is trying to think about. And how can that be, he wonders, as he sinks deeper in his chair, when he has always loved to think? How can that be, when he has always been so good at it?

He has been called a great thinker. Gazing at the odd set of old hands lying slack in his lap, he remembers hearing that very phrase used to describe him while he waits, stiff with worry and breathless from his recent sprint, in the wings of the auditorium at the University of London, listening with less than half an ear as the president of the International Shakespeare Society lists his achievements for the benefit of the assembled crowd.

He spent all summer working on that speech, first rereading Plutarch and Erasmus and Foucault, then revisiting all the critics whose insights he valued most, and finally sketching out endless drafts of his own ideas, patiently balancing his condemnations with concessions, trying to make his address more entertaining and more persuasive than anything he'd ever written before.

He has looked forward to this moment for many months, but now he wishes it were already over, now he wonders if he should be standing there at all. When his hearing snags on those words—*great thinker*—he is momentarily startled to realize that it is to him the president is referring. He wishes he could allow himself even a moment to bask in her praise. But instead he is tearing through his briefcase one more time, searching for the speech he knows is still sitting on the nightstand back in his hotel room.

And now he pauses in his frantic, fruitless search to peer around the heavy velvet curtain and scan the audience for its most unlikely member. But although he spots Freya, sitting on the aisle in her raw silk suit, her legs crossed at the thigh and a pump dangling from one foot as if boredom were her biggest problem at that moment, he can locate no purple-haired teenager among that staid crowd.

Suddenly, the president is calling out his name and the audience is responding as if Dr. John Wilson were a rock star instead of a Shakespearean scholar. Behind the dusty curtain he snatches a breath for luck and inspiration, but as he propels himself out into the lights and applause, he feels a surge of fury to think that this golden chance has been ruined so entirely by his daughter.

He wants to weep. Sitting in his worn chair, he wants to press his face into his hands and weep until tears pour like rivers between his fingers. No, he wants to roar. He wants to roar until the green walls fall, until the very air bursts into flame. He wants to weep and roar and rage. Like Lear, he wants the thunder of his passion to strike flat the thick rotundity of the world. Like Othello, he wants to put out every light.

Fury surges in his limbs, welcome as an orgasm for the way it helps to quell his sorrows. He wants to hurt the world, to make it bleed. He wants to raze the calm linoleum, smash the window, rip up the quiet turf. There is a chair next to his own, and it infuriates him, that chair. Both its presence and the absence it suggests offend him in some keen way. He is angry at that chair, and angrier still that he can't say why. With a roar, he rises from his own seat, attacks that scurrilous chair, and flings it to the ground.

But its little clatter is too empty, its fall too meager to leave him satisfied. Askew upon the floor, it seems more like a reproach than an achievement.

He turns his passion to the other chair, the larger, hide-clad one. Grabbing its back with both his hands, he shifts his weight, tries to throw it down. Straining like a wrestler, he growls and grunts, fighting until the tendons in his hands stand out like knives. But even with his anger as a fulcrum, the chair remains upright.

It seems such a simple thing, to topple a chair. But in the end, trembling with chagrin and unspent rage, he sinks back into its implacable lap instead. Groaning, his chest heaving with effort and frustration, he bends his face toward his knees, cradles his head in his hands, sits huddled and inert as stone. All his life he has been bright, quick, keen, intelligent. His mind has been an engine, a falcon, a beacon, an open door. Never before have his brains abandoned him.

"Hey, John." A woman pops into the room like a well-rehearsed bit player, lacking only the letter or the lance that would justify her appearance onstage. Her name begins with a hum. Or a moan.

"What happened here?" she tuts, round arms akimbo as she looks from him to the chair upended on the floor. Bending over, she rights it, then groans and jams her hand into the small of her back as she straightens up.

"They're having a party down in the day lounge to celebrate the July birthdays. You wanna go?" she asks, reaching down to place her plump hand on his old boned one.

"No," he answers, the word a stone.

"There'll be cake and ice cream," the woman cajoles. In the sky above his walled green world, new clouds are gathering. When he does not reply, she teases, "Aw, come on. Give it a try."

"I'm busy."

"Give it a chance," the woman urges, "it might be fun."

"Fun, nothing," he answers. "I don't have time for . . ." he says, but though he gropes around inside his mind, he cannot find the word he wants. "Fun," he adds feebly.

"Are you sure?" Concern warming her tone, she suggests, "I keep thinking you'd be happier if you got involved more, maybe made some friends." The drench of her care is tempting. But he's learned about such sweet traps, he's seen firsthand the emptiness inside. And besides, he thinks contemptuously, there is no *fun* in Shakespeare. It's not a word he had, nor one he ever felt the need to coin. For Shakespeare, *joy, delight,* and *happiness* sufficed.

"Okay," she answers with a melodramatic sigh, "just be that way."

From down the hall comes the sound of "Happy Birthday" being sung. John hears the voluble piano, hears the thin ribbon of old people singing, their voices lagging behind the brisk notes.

He remembers singing "Happy Birthday"—singing, and then watching as a girl of nine or ten expands her skinny chest and puffs her cheeks to gust out the candles on the cake in front of her. He remembers how the sheen of her pleasure seems like another flame, how, despite the tensions that fill the candlelit darkness of that dining room, his heart balloons at the sight of that child's happiness.

Her birthday always came at an awkward time—three days after Christmas, right at the start of the Modern Language Association's yearly convention. Back when he was still married to Barb, it had been easier to make sure there were gifts and balloons and a cake whose candles he could witness Miranda extinguishing—either before he left for the conference or after he returned. But once he and Barb had parted, and especially after he left Santa Cruz for a more prestigious position at a less prestigious university three hours north, it became harder to make sure her birthday was adequately remembered.

The winter after the London debacle, he was still trying to decide how he should react to her foul-mouthed rejection when her birthday arrived. Ever since his disastrous visit back in September he'd expected that she would get in touch with him. He had even been rehearsing the words he would use to forgive her when she did. He understood she'd been more hurt than he'd expected by his decision to send her home, and he'd thought he should give her space to regain her equilibrium. But when Christmas came and went without his having heard from her, he began to worry their impasse had gone on too long.

He had not had the easiest of times himself that autumn. He'd received nothing but rejections—with no invitations for resubmission—to the article he'd developed from his ISS speech, none of the presses he'd queried about editing an anthology on revitalizing the humanities had even responded, and he hadn't been asked to review a single chapter, book, or article all fall. When Freya began to sleep in the guest bedroom after they returned from Spain, he'd assumed at first it was because of her book deadline, but after she sent off her manuscript and still did not return to his bed, he finally had to admit which way that wind was blowing.

It distressed him no end to think his third marriage was nearing its final act. He'd left one woman he shouldn't have left, and another he should never have married, and now a woman he probably should not have married appeared to be leaving him. Freya had seemed so right when they were wooing—not only brilliant and in his field, but also comely and young. He'd been proud—and even faintly astounded—by her interest in him. But now it appeared that he'd been even more of a trophy for her than she had been for him. He'd helped to open some hefty doors for her while she was finishing her PhD and trying to place her book. But as soon as she'd started opening doors herself, she began to dismiss his ideas as plodding and sentimental, to complain about his Eurocentric bias and his privileging of certain worn-out texts.

Over the holidays, he'd begun to hope her feelings were starting to thaw. On their flight to Dallas where the conference was being held that year, he even dared to think he spied in her high spirits some marks of love returning, though as soon as they arrived at the convention center, he was disappointed when she staked out the desk in their hotel room, and began rehearsing for her Harvard interview with the single-minded focus of a presidential candidate prepping for her final debate.

He hung around their room that first afternoon in a dilatory way, trying to do some work himself, but also stewing about his daughter's unbroken silence and his wife's ongoing reserve.

"I'm trying to decide what to do about Miranda," he confessed, when, after several hours, Freya finally took a break to use the bathroom. He was interested in her insights as a former teenaged girl, though he was also half imagining that if she were to offer any advice—and especially if he employed it—she might become more invested in the entire situation than she had been heretofore.

"What about her?" she snapped.

"Today's her birthday, and I haven't heard from her all fall—not since she was so rude to me. I'm trying to decide whether I should get in touch with her now or not."

"She called that one time," Freya offered absently.

"What? What one time? When?"

"I told you," she answered, bending back over the new laptop computer of which she was so proud.

"No, you didn't. I never heard a word."

"I'm sure I did. You must have forgotten. She was rude to me, too."

"I wouldn't have forgotten that. When did she call? What did she say?" He didn't want to add to the gulf between them by unfairly blaming Freya for anything, but it was hard to temper his alarm.

"She just said she wanted to talk to you." Freya lifted her head to glare at him. "A month or so ago. She didn't say why. She hung up on me as soon as I said you weren't home. I know I told you about it, though if I forgot, I'm sorry. But really, it was probably just a passing whim. If it meant all that much to her, she would have called back.

"Anyway," she added with a shrug, "if you want to talk to her, by all means go ahead and call."

After Freya left to meet her dissertation advisor for a predinner drink, he waited nearly an hour until he calculated that Miranda would be home from school, and then he placed the call.

Her hello held that breathless mix of hope and hesitance with which so many teenaged girls answer the phone. Hearing it, he'd been suffused by such a flood of sympathy and love it seemed that every sour memory was instantly washed away. She had so much promise, he thought, she was still so young. Her escapades in London were evidence of a kid with spunk, with spark. And if hearing her tell him to fuck off had come as a cruel shock, maybe it was important somehow, too, as another level of honesty, a new rite of passage. He had never had that kind of clarity with his own father. Perhaps if he'd had, they would not have ended up such strangers to each other.

"Happy birthday," he announced.

"Thanks," she answered warily, all the bright expectation having drained from her voice the instant she heard his.

"Are you having a good one?"

"I guess."

"I can't believe you're seventeen already," he observed, though the moment the words were out of his mouth, he could hear how wrong they were.

"Well, well. How about that?" Her voice was a parody of his, the fake cheer of it so acid it seemed it might corrode the phone line.

"I wanted to tell you happy birthday," he persisted, "but I also wanted you to know that I've missed you this fall. I've hated to be out of touch."

"Yeah. Well."

"I think you called," he plunged on, "a couple of months ago. Freya must have forgotten to give me the message, and I'm really sorry. I had no idea. I only just found out. If I'd known, of course I would have called you right—"

But at that moment, Freya entered the room, scowling to find him on the phone.

"—back," he finished, suddenly reluctant to risk vexing his wife by pursuing that topic any further.

"Anyway," he added a little awkwardly as Freya bent toward the mirror above the washstand alcove and began to sleek her hair and brush fresh blush along her cheekbones. "I wondered, did you have anything specific you wanted to talk about?"

"No," she said curtly.

"Really?" He waited another beat, and when she didn't offer anything more, he asked, "Well, how're you doing now? Did you have a good Christmas?"

"It was okay."

"What did you do?"

"Nothing."

"Nothing?"

"Christmas crap," she said sharply.

The insolence of her tone kindled in him an unexpected flicker of the fury and frustration he'd known when the smirking bobbies who'd found her asleep at the base of one of the lions in Trafalgar Square delivered her—pale and teetering and reeking of booze—back to the hotel, observing that although she'd refused to reveal much about what she'd done or where she'd been, p'raps it weren't too hard to read between the lines?

Trying to override those recollections, he asked, "Everything going okay in school?"

"I dropped out."

"Dropped out?" he gasped, while Freya narrowed her eyes at the mirror and gave herself a complacent little nod. "Your mother never told me. When?"

"Before Thanksgiving."

"What were you think—"

"April Fools," she interjected.

"Oh," he said with a spatter of uneasy laughter. Nodding at Freya's signal that she was headed out to meet their group for dinner, he added, "I get it—joke?"

"You really don't know, do you?" she said, disgust twisting her words. "You have no idea whether I'm joking or not."

"I'm trying to find out," he answered evenly as Freya closed the door. "I'm trying to talk to you—right now—to see how you're doing. I can't possibly know how you're doing unless you tell me, Miranda."

"I'm Randi," she announced belligerently. "That's my name."

"You do know—don't you?—that in England 'randy' means—" He paused, suddenly reluctant to define the word to his own daughter. "Lascivious," he added a beat later.

"And you do know—don't you?—that this is America? And whatever the fuck 'lascivious' means, well, maybe that's exactly what I am."

"Miran—"

"I'm through with this shit—get it? You call me when it's convenient for you, and then you expect me to be your perfect little paper doll princess—'happy birthday,' 'how was Christmas?' bla, bla, bla. Well, fuck you all over again. Just fuck you. I never want to talk to you again."

Afterwards, instead of joining Freya and their supper group, he'd lain on the massive bed, staring at the ceiling and straining to trace the demise of his relationship with his daughter, to pinpoint where things had veered so wrong. But when he tried to determine what he might have done differently, the answer he arrived at was both everything and nothing at all, and when he tried to consider how he should proceed now, the only thought that came to him was that it might be wise to sort things out with Freya before he tried to contact Miranda again.

At supper, John suffers the roast beef, green salad, and mashed potato on his plate while the clown across from him claims a magician walking down the street turned into a bar, and the stout woman at his side warbles about a surrey with a fringe on top, and some beldame at another table weeps as if she has forgotten how to stop.

"E flat walks into a bar," the long-jawed churl announces, "and the bartender tells him, 'Sorry, we don't serve minors.' Shakespeare walks into a bar, and the bartender says, 'We can't serve you—you're bard here.'"

When John returns to the room that has somehow become a kind of sorry home, he resumes his watch at the window, gazing through the shadowy glass at the darkening wall and pale sky. There is so much that hurts him, so much he doesn't understand. He has been wronged so many ways, has been thwarted and blighted and sorely abused.

It is the size of the characters' desires that helps to make a sad story a tragedy. John tells his students that. In the face of all life's niggling and haggling, despite all the disappointments and petty outrages that train most humans to smallness, Shakespeare's heroes' desires burn bright, demanding that the world make an answer.

But when the answer comes, it comes too late. He tells his students that, too. In his classes he explains that tragedy's most cruel lesson is not that human beings are flawed, or that fate can be unkind, but that no one can ever slip the bonds of time.

Outside, the dark is deepening. Above the wall a single star shines in the cobalt air. Remote, unerring, silent, it provokes in John a yearning that twists his heart. *Bright particular star,* he thinks as he studies it, and, *yond same star   not in the stars, But in ourselves   Some consequence yet hanging in the stars   Take him and cut him out in little stars*

162

Anon another memory brims in him, and once again he sits in his office in the English department in Michigan, listening as a student recites Juliet's lines about cutting Romeo into little stars.

She is in his intro class, a senior finishing up her last general ed requirement. He'd spotted her on the first day, watching quietly from the back of the room as he strutted and fretted his hour in the lecture hall, creating the persona that would carry him through the semester—iconoclastic professor, scrupulous scholar, fervent apostle of William Shakespeare.

That first morning, he'd noted her blond hair and creamy arms, the way her breasts stood out from her chest like a second opinion. She was yet another instance of the fresh and luscious coed, but even more than her shiny new beauty or the untapped intelligence he thought he spied in her soft brown eyes, John found himself perversely intrigued by her very lack of receptivity to his professorial charm. While her classmates smiled at his mildest joke and nodded to signal their rapt attention to his merest word, she studied his performance coolly, as if she were immune to both message and messenger.

For the next half semester she hovered at the edge of his imagination, half inspiration and half goad. Often her image appeared in his mind while he planned his lectures, and sometimes in the classroom he realized he was doing what he understood that actors did when they attempted to strengthen their performances by choosing one member of the audience on which to focus their delivery. But despite the extra energy his awareness of her lent his lectures, she remained on the margin of the class, taking notes but never actually offering anything herself.

Because he had a graduate assistant to grade his students' papers, he did not actually speak with her or even learn her name until one raw-winded day in early November when, as he was walking back to his office after class, he heard someone running to catch up with him.

"Professor Wilson?" Although he had yet to hear her speak, even before he turned to see her sprinting up the walkway he knew it was she.

"Can I talk with you a sec?" she gasped, breathless from the cold wind and her run. "I can never make it to your office hours because I have other classes."

Her disheveled hair was spread across her face like a shining veil, and for a moment John's impulse to brush it back into place was so strong that even in his distant cell, his hand twitches in his lap, remembering.

"Talk away," he answered with a flourish of his arm as if he were an actor playing a courtier instead of an associate professor of English. Beneath her open coat she clutched her books to her chest so that they raised and flattened her breasts like an Elizabethan bodice. Suddenly, the bone-chilling wind seemed invigorating. Glancing past her, John saw how the leaves of the ivy clinging to the building they stood beside fluttered like scarlet pennants in the wind.

Falling in next to him, she explained that she had never before read Shakespeare, that she was having lots more trouble than she'd expected. In fact, even though it would set back her graduation date, she was thinking of dropping John's course. Bending her head like a swan as they pushed side by side into the stinging wind, she confessed, "I didn't get hardly anything out of *Twelfth Night* or *Richard II*, and now that we've started *Romeo and Juliet*, I don't understand a quarter of that play, either. And when I do get it—honestly, it's mainly just a bunch of clichés—'wherefore art thou Romeo?' 'parting is such sweet sorrow.'" She spoke a little timorously, as if she were reluctant to criticize, and yet committed to saying what she saw to be the truth. "All his people ever do is talk."

Her name was Barbara. Gazing up at that bright star, John thinks that even if he hadn't been beguiled by her face and breasts and the hair that blew like tangled silk across her lips, he would still have tried to find a way to convert her. In the tavern where graduate students and professors gathered to gossip about grants and deans and complain about the ignorance or the indifference of their students, he always came to the students' defense. It was urgent to reach them, he argued, barbaric as they might first appear, both for the sake of civilization, as well as for their own inchoate souls.

"Exactly!" he answered her now, punching the cold wind with a triumphant fist. "Don't you see?—you're already under his spell! What did you just say? 'All his people ever do is talk.' *His* people. His *people*. Stop for a minute to think about that." Pausing in front of the building that housed his office, he turned to face her while groups of students hurried past, their faces buried in their jackets. "Shakespeare's characters are not people. They do not bleed or cry. Romeo and Juliet never died. Mercutio never scoffed at love. All they are is ideas, just little strings of sounds, little packages of words. *They* don't talk—they *are* talk. Just marks on a page or voices on a stage, and yet already you're thinking of them as people—human beings just like you and me—people who can bicker and suffer, think and fight, and," he paused for the merest sliver of a second before the wind whipped the word from his lips, "love.

"Stick with it," he urged, allowing himself a brief, professorial pat on the sleeve of her coat. "Keep reading. You're obviously more than bright enough, and I suspect you have more than enough heart. It'll start to make sense, I promise. Think of reading Shakespeare as listening to a very wise and fun—and funny—friend with a foreign accent. At first it can be a challenge to understand what someone like that is saying. But once you get to know him better, you'll hardly notice his accent. And later you'll come to love how much the way he says something adds to everything he says. Don't give up," he added with a sage smile. "And in the meantime, if you have more questions, don't hesitate to let me know."

And suddenly he is complicit, already in too far. He sees that now, and he wonders why he could not see it then. Looking back from this far lip of time, John feels a terrible shiver of foreboding, a tinge of shame, another knife's twist of pain. He aches to caution that former self—*his* former self, he supposes, though the connection between them perplexes him, and he cannot comprehend why he should have to accept as his a self so remote and inexplicable, so beyond his control.

He'd had a wife back then, the wife he'd met as an undergraduate at UC Davis and married the week after they graduated. They'd given their virginities to each other a month before their wedding, and although the act itself had been more awkward than sublime, it had felt both right and worldly to consummate their marriage before they consecrated it.

That wife had put him through graduate school by teaching history to eighth and ninth graders. She moved with him to Michigan when he was offered the job there, and now that he is tenured and well on his way to becoming the youngest full professor in the department, she wants them to begin a family. She wants him to travel with her during their vacations instead of spending his time on articles or conference presentations. She doesn't like it when he stops by the tavern to argue about the meaning of nothing or the salvation of freshmen instead of coming home to her. She wants more attention from him, more affection—though lately she's taken to complaining how every hug or snuggle turns his mind toward sex.

Even so, he assumes he loves her—or at least feels for her a complex mix of habit and tenderness, duty and gratitude that much resembles love. And so he is unprepared when he opens his office door a few days later to find Barbara standing outside in the hall, a few melted drops from the season's first snowfall clinging to her hair like living jewels.

For a second he assumes she has come to continue the conversation it suddenly seems he's been having with her inside his head all fall. But the hesitant way she stands in the doorway recalls him to his senses, and he invites her in like the courteous professor that he is. She is wearing a pair of leather hot pants over maroon tights and a maroon turtleneck, and when she sits in the chair he offers her, he rations glances at the lean lines of her thighs.

"It's *Romeo and Juliet*," she announces. "I just finished reading it."

"Really?" he answers. "And?"

"I don't know what happened, but suddenly it was like it just kind of clicked for me. It's beautiful, really. So sweet." Shaking her head at the memory, she adds, "So sad."

"What makes you call it sad?" he asks. And holds his breath.

"What makes it sad?" She scrunches her lovely brow. "How alone they are, I guess," she answers slowly. "That no one else in Verona understood the total goodness of their love. Well, maybe the Friar did." She pauses, tilting her head to one side as if she were listening to her own thoughts. "Though even he wasn't willing to just let their love exist. He wanted to use it, too—to try to get their families back together."

"You're thinking well," John answers, leaning back in his chair— expansive, casual, in control. "What's the question you think I might be able to help you with?"

"It's probably dumb," she offers shyly. "I mean, I'm sure it is."

"There's no such thing as a dumb question," he answers gallantly. And in that moment he actually believes it.

"When Juliet says, you know . . . those lines about cutting Romeo into little stars?"

"Yes?"

"It's just that I recognized them. At least, I thought I did."

"Really?" John asks, leaning forward.

"My dad was a colonel in the Air Force, but his plane got shot down." She speaks neutrally, looking not at John but into another world entirely— some near and distant place he suddenly fears he may never reach.

"I'm sorry." Leaning forward, he asks, "In Vietnam?"

"Khe Sanh." She shifts her gaze from that other world back to him, looking at him as if she were seeing him for the first time.

He shakes his head at the many sorrows of it—an able man killed, a woman bereft of her husband, a daughter entering adulthood without her father, the waste and horror of the war John is of course opposed to. But before he can form the right response, she says, "My mom wanted those words carved on his headstone. She'd heard Bobby Kennedy say them for his brother, some time or other. She was pretty broke up when she found out it would cost too much to put them on Dad's marker."

She gives herself a quick hug, squeezing her maroon-clad arms across her chest so that her exquisite breasts rise even higher. "I don't think she even knew that Shakespeare wrote it, but I recognized that part when I read the play.

"'Give me my Romeo,'" she says, looking shyly into some sweeter distance,

> "'and when I shall die,
> Take him and cut him out in little stars,
> And he will make the face of heaven so fine
> that all the world will be in love with night,
> and pay no worship to the garish sun.'"

She seems embarrassed to be speaking those lines aloud, but below her discomfort John can hear the irrepressible lilt of the poetry, the natural music of her voice. He sits a moment, basking in the beauty of the words, savoring the little thrill it gives him to hear her speak them to him—even so obliquely.

"You've memorized that!" he says to break a silence that suddenly threatens to grow too deep.

"It wasn't hard," she answers with another lovely shrug. "Only," she adds tentatively, "Here's what I don't understand. Isn't it supposed to be, 'When *he* shall die'? Not *I*—not Juliet dying—but *he*—Romeo?

"I keep thinking that Mom must of got confused, because what she wanted on Dad's headstone is not the way it says it in our book. But then that's confusing, too, because it doesn't make any sense—does it?—for Mom to want to put it on Dad's headstone if it says, 'when I shall die,' since Dad's the one that's gone. It's like the—whatsit?—the point of view is wrong. Why would Juliet want Romeo to be chopped into pieces when *she* dies? I mean, what if Romeo's still alive?"

Nodding gravely, John lets a moment pass in silent appreciation of her question before he speaks. "Back when I first began to study *Romeo and Juliet*, the pronoun in the second clause of the twenty-first line of act three, scene two of all the standard editions of the play was *he*. It wasn't until I was in graduate school that I ran across an edition that used *I* instead, and when I did, I was sure I'd found a misprint. In fact," he adds, indulging a wry smile intended to express both fondness and condescension for the ambitious, untutored student he'd once been, "for a few seconds I even imagined I was going to earn a little glory for having caught an error."

"Yeah?" she says, watching him intently. "I mean—yes?"

"But it turns out that the only original text that uses *he* is the Fourth Quarto, which is a late and otherwise unauthoritative reprinting of the third. There's no reason to think the changes that appear in that Quarto are anything other than a typesetter's attempt to tidy up what he saw as errors in the previous printings. Because the fact is, that in every other Quarto—and in the Folio, too—Juliet says, 'when I shall die.' And so we must assume that is what Shakespeare intended."

"But that changes everything," she bursts out indignantly. "It changes the whole play."

"And how does it do that?" he asks, suddenly warmed by a nearly paternal pride.

"It's one thing if Juliet wanted him cut into little pieces after he'd already died. It's like she thought he was so perfect that even after he was dead he could still decorate the whole universe." She stops for a moment, tilting her head to one side in the charming gesture John has already learned signals that she is thinking. "And maybe," she continues slowly, as if she were in the process of discovering her thought as she speaks it, "maybe after he's dead, she'd be willing to share him with the world—*her* Romeo.

"But it just seems so selfish, for her to want him hacked to pieces when *she* dies. It reminds me of those things in India—what're they called?—where the wife gets burned alive along with her dead husband."

"Suttee?" John offers. "Though in this case I suppose the sexes would have to be reversed."

"Yeah." She shudders. "That's so creepy. Juliet never loved Romeo like that."

"In the balcony scene, she does say she might kill him with much cherishing," John suggests. He is touched by her fervency, moved by her romanticism, thrilled by what he perceives as her raw intelligence. Despite his own increasing cynicism about *Romeo and Juliet*, he suddenly finds himself hoping that she will stand up for that other, older, more innocent vision of the play.

"Kill him with much cherishing?" she echoes. She looks puzzled for a moment, and then she says, "You mean like that bird on a string thing?"

"A silken thread, yes," John answers, watching spellbound as her thoughts move like patterns of sun and shadow across her face.

"But isn't that different? Isn't she saying that's what she wouldn't want to do—kill him with much cherishing?"

"Could be." John pauses for a moment before asking, "What do you make of the fact that she's thinking about dying from practically the moment she first meets Romeo? 'If he be married, My grave is like to be my wedding bed,' is what she says after she's exchanged less than half a dozen lines with the guy. After that, dying is never far from her thoughts. In fact, we might say her anticipation of death saturates the whole play."

"Maybe she's willing to die for her love," Barbara answers, "but I can't believe she wants Romeo to be killed."

"There's one more thing for you to consider," John says gravely, "yet another fact scholars have found germane to this particular question. And that is, that for the Elizabethans—and certainly for Shakespeare— one meaning of 'to die' was to experience sexual ecstasy."

"Se—?" she begins, and then catches herself, as if startled to be on the verge of blurting such a phrase in a professor's office.

"As I've pointed out in class, Shakespeare explores all of human experience, including the totality of love, and one way some scholars have had of understanding Juliet's line is in a sexual context."

Despite her blush, it suddenly seems that some bold new understanding has appeared in her expression, a discovery or a calculation far removed from the additional definition of a word. For a moment they sit together in an odd charged silence, and then, when it appears she has nothing more to ask about the play, John stands to see her to the door. Offering her a grave smile, he says, "I think you've discovered a promising topic for your term paper, and I'll be more than happy to help you work on it if you'd like. If my office hours aren't convenient for you, perhaps we can make other arrangements."

What was he thinking, who had he been? he wonders now as further stars appear in the blackening sky. Who was that foolish man who was so unable to interpret a character, discern a motive, or even predict a plot? *What's done cannot be undone.* It's Lady Macbeth who makes that mournful claim, though she is talking about the murder of a king, nothing so trivial as John's offer to help a coed study Shakespeare. But even so, the stage is set, the great wheel turns, already the charm is firm and good.

He yearns to return to the cramped office where that previous John sits admiring that coed's lovely thighs, yearns to warn that dotard of his impending folly. He wishes he could smash the bond of time, break the fourth wall—or maybe the fourth dimension—and speak directly to that earlier self. He would tell him to be wary, would remind him that all that glisters is not gold, that his heart is already a tangled web.

But you cannot communicate with the past, despite its being prologue to every now. All those other men that John has been—they can talk to him, but he cannot speak back to them.

"John, John, John," a woman clucks. "What are you doing, sitting in the dark?" He hears a click and light stabs his eyes as the clucker whisks on down the hall. Suddenly the window has become a black mirror, his own face masking his view of whatever is going on beyond the glass. But surely little lives continue in that garden all night long—the unseen worms and voles and crows doing whatever their kind do when the sun is gone, the hungry snails, the sleeping bees, the dreaming butterflies. The silent stars still shining. Entire universes spiraling beyond his ken while John strains to see the world—or even himself—through his own reflected eyes.

"You can't see beyond your own dick!" Nancy had shrieked. Though to her credit, she'd shrieked it only once. Otherwise, their demise had been as civil as such a disunion can be—more tears than accusations, more silent suffering than angry battles. Poor Nancy. John hadn't realized how heartsick she would be when he told her he was leaving. He'd been in such a froth himself, so smitten with the lovely novelty of Barbara that he'd assumed there was no real substance to their marriage for Nancy either, that beneath the veneer of their partnership there existed only a little desiccated affection.

But it seemed to have worked all right for Nancy in the end. Eighteen months after their divorce was finalized, she married the biology teacher at the high school where she taught, and they'd had two children in quick succession. John saw her once years later, when he'd been back in

Chicago for some conference or other. They met for a cocktail in the bar of the convention center, and when she showed him photographs of her son in his West Point uniform and her daughter cradling her first baby, there'd been the briefest instant when John assumed those people were somehow related to him, too. A moment later, an image of his own sullen daughter entered his mind, and although it added to his envy of Nancy's clean-cut brood, he'd also known an odd sense of superiority to think his child was not such a sheep.

Nancy. She'd seemed so drab when he was succumbing to Barbara's excellent witchcraft. But she'd looked good in that cocktail lounge. Sitting opposite her in the bar's deep booth, he'd been flooded with a montage of memories from their marriage, and he'd known a sharp regret.

He hears a woman weeping. In the strange and vivid theater inside his mind he sees her, too—Barbara, sobbing among the tangled sheets. Sitting in his worn chair, John stands in the doorway of that long-gone bedroom and watches as she cries.

It's a scene too tawdry to be a tragedy. From his empty helm in this dimming room, he sees all the sorry meagerness of that moment, and standing in the doorway of what has been their mutual bedchamber, he sees it, too, senses both the futility of the present and the finality of the future he has just made possible bearing down on him. He feels a gut stab of remorse, a million prickles of regret. He yearns for some other, easier way.

As Barb lies sobbing into her hands on the bed that John has not shared for many a night, he wonders yet again if he is right to be leaving her. He wonders if it might not be possible to fix things, even now. Maybe he could find a way to make this not an ending but a new—and truer—start.

It's not Barb's fault she knows herself so little, not her fault she is incapable of matching John anywhere but in bed. It is arguably not even her fault she's begun to dabble in adultery, taking it up like yoga or needlepoint, a hobby to keep herself occupied while he is working and Miranda is off at school. He has made this mistake once before, leaving a woman he did not really have to leave. Maybe this time he just needs grit enough to sleep in the bed he's made, guts enough to stay with this weeping woman, wisdom enough to trust that time will teach the two of them what true love is.

He knows that one word—or two or three—are all the moment will require, knows the real work will come later, and though he wastes a fleet second in wishing that Shakespeare had had more to say about living—instead of wedding or dying—in the service of love, in that second he believes he could surely find a way to do that, too.

Already anticipating the relief of reconciliation, he makes a step toward the bed while Barb lowers her hands to peek at him over the pickets of her pink-tipped fingernails. Even brimming with tears, her eyes are lovely, and John takes another, swifter step, ready to melt into their melting. But now a flicker of calculation enters her expression. Covering her face again, she continues to weep, though John senses she is also gathering resources, calculating strategies, deciding with all the self-conscious skill of an accomplished actress or a master rhetorician exactly how she will react when he touches her, precisely what she will concede and what demand.

A vision of their future life together sweeps over him, the endless dreary days of boredom and capitulation, the constant concessions for Miranda's sake, his daily calculations about whether it will be harder on Miranda to have to hear her parents quarrel yet again or to witness him giving in once more to her mother's narcissistic whims.

When John does not join her on the bed, Barb sneaks another glance. In that instant she seems to recognize he is not coming, that he will never come again, and some precariously balanced power comes crashing down, exploding like his mother's antique ginger jar when Barb flung it across the living room the week before. He is turning to walk out of the room when she rises off the bed to hiss, "You can take everything else—and I know you will. But I'll never let you have Miranda."

As John descends the stairs, he contemplates this new threat. He has always assumed that, like the other divorced parents he knows, he and Barb would work out some equitable way of sharing the remaining years of Miranda's childhood. If anything, he's expected Barb would welcome the chance for Miranda to spend more time with him while she pursued her amorous adventures unimpeded. Barb has never been very motherly, and lately she's seemed more bored than adoring of her daughter.

But maybe, John ponders as he reaches the landing, he's been wrong about that. Maybe Miranda means more to Barb than John has been aware. And if parenting Miranda is what Barb needs, then perhaps it would be in everyone's best interests if he let that happen. He knows compromise is important. Despite Barb's accusations, he wants what's fair. He has never expected to have everything. He wants what's best for Miranda, first of all.

But now the sound of weeping has stopped. John hears water running in the bathroom, and he realizes if he doesn't leave the house before Barb comes downstairs, they will be embroiled yet again. He tells himself he needs to be stoic, needs to finish cleanly what was so messily begun. He knows it has been hard on Miranda, to have to watch her parents snipe and bicker for so long. She needs to see adults being reasonable, finding ways to get along. Despite the fact that it's dull Polonius's pompous platitude, he wants her to see how important it is to be true to her own self.

When he hears Barb call his name, he opens the door and steps outside into the damp afternoon. It isn't as if he will never see Miranda again, he reasons, as he walks away. Even if she ends up living with her mother, Barb will surely want weekends off. Besides, don't girls need their mothers? How could he give Miranda the help with tampons and proms, bras and boyfriends he knows she will need in the next few years? All will be well, he promises himself as he climbs into his car. In the end, everything will work out just fine.

But he was wrong about that, too, John thinks, staring beyond the black glass of the window he sits facing and back into that hapless past. Nothing worked out at all. He waited for years, and a better ending never came.

"It's time for bed," a gentle voice suggests.

A slight, dark woman stands beside him, holding a folded pile of fabric between her outstretched hands as if she were offering him a gift. "Here are your pajamas, Mistah Wilson." Her voice lilts with an accented English that seems more kin to music than to speech as she helps him stand, helps him find his way out of his shirt and slacks and socks and underclothes, helps him fit himself into the pajamas. In the bathroom she hands him a toothbrush, and when he is finished, gives him a warm washcloth with which to wipe his face.

Once he is flat in bed with the covers tucked around him, she lays her delicate hand against his blanketed chest. "Good night," she says after a quiet moment.

Sleep tight, his mother's voice answers as the woman slips from the room, the ghostly iamb of her words echoing down the decades to reach John where he lies swaddled in bedclothes and nightclothes, gazing at the light streaming through the open door.

But his mother is gone.

He remembers. She left him in another century, rode away in the front seat of the Packard in her good wool suit. She's gone forever now, she's dead as earth. When he and Sally visited her grave in the pioneer cemetery outside of Kernville, the letters on the granite marker that spelled her name were already softening with the grinding of the years, as if the stone itself were learning to forget her.

Sally's gone, too.

Or at least she's not here now—now, when he misses her so urgently it is as if she were some essential organ he is suddenly expected to survive without. He misses her muscled arms and the sunny crinkles around her eyes, misses the friendly press of her soft breasts as he lays him down to sleep beside her. A wife like a gift, a benison beyond his deserving, a wife with beauty in her eye, since, as he is fond of reminding her, beauty is in the eye of the bee holder.

He'd agreed to the mazy plan that led him to this lonely bed because he wanted to ease her worries, wanted anything that pains her to go away. He'd agreed because he loves her, because he pledged his life and troth to her, because he was so loath to fail at marriage one more time.

Back when he first found Sally and was realizing her worth, he thought he'd been given a chance as golden and unearned as any that graced the endings of Shakespeare's romances. When, borrowing the words from Prince Florizel, he'd told her, *I cannot be Mine own, nor any thing to any, if I be not thine,* tears had graced her eyes. She'd taken his crabbed hand in her dear calloused one and kissed the hollow at his temple that she claimed to love, and in that moment he'd truly believed a world had been redeemed. At their wedding, he'd said that he and she were like the single pair of eyes which, working together, gives vision its depth.

He thought he had been blessed with a joy as hard-won and undeserved as that of the precious winners in *The Winter's Tale*. He'd believed his sixth act, too, would be a happy one. But he'd been too old to play Prince Florizel, John thinks with a hot fierce flush. He'd learned how love works long ago. "Sonnet 116" and bearing it out even to the edge of doom notwithstanding, he'd understood for over half a century that there is no evil angel but love.

Love is a dream from which one wakes older but no better, wiser only in sorrows. Love fades. Or rots. Or never really was. Or if there were a sympathy in choice, war, death, or sickness did lay siege to it.

The course of true love never did run smooth; he remembers chanting out that line from *A Midsummer Night's Dream* for some small child, a girl of six or eight, who, sitting on his lap, laps up his words. Studying his lips with her brown eyes, she frowns and listens, nods in time to his recital, and then repeats the lines herself, occasionally getting stuck until he leans in to whisper what comes next as if they were sharing the breaking of a rule.

He feels again the delicious warmth of her slight weight, sees again how she strains, squinching up her face as if she might squeeze the lines from her brain like toothpaste, while he nods his encouragement, circling his hands as if to coax the next words from her. He remembers his delight when she announces she is ready to recite the whole speech, remembers how she begins as intently as a long-distance runner, and then, when it is clear the end is in sight, how she breaks into a wide, proud smile as she chants the final lines:

"'Or if there were a sympathy in choice,
War, death, or sickness did lay siege to it,
Making it momentary as a sound
Swift as a shadow, short as any dream
Brief as the lightening in the collied night,
That, in a spleen, unfolds both heaven and earth;
And ere a man hath power to say "Behold!"
The jaws of darkness do devour it up:
So quick bright things come to confusion.'"

"Brava!" he cries when she is finished. Snatching up her hand, he pumps it in the air. Reaching down beside his chair for their box of Cracker Jack, he fills the doubled cup of her palms with caramel kernels.

"'So quick bright things come to confusion.'" Lying stiff as grief in his single bed, John listens as that ghost-girl lisps those lambent words. Her mouth is not yet hard enough to pronounce the *r* in *bright*, the *th* sound in *things*. He knows another surge of pride at her precociousness, though at the same time he feels a pinch of remorse at the pessimism in the lines he is teaching her. *The jaws of darkness do devour it up*—he wishes he might somehow protect her from that doleful fact—*swift as a shadow, short as any dream*

And yet it is the truth. Even in the comedies the characters know that. Love comes to confusion. Always. And so quick. And not just love, but all bright things—every shine and spark, each pulse and hope and effort—everything extinguished, lost or squandered. *So quick bright things*

Even Shakespeare came to confusion, John reflects bitterly, when he wrote his final plays—those foppish romances with which he ended his career. Once, John had planned to end his own career as their champion. Until quite lately he had believed the romances were evidence of some brave new vision, proof of art's power, of humanity's capacity for grace and growth.

But tonight he agrees with all those other critics—whose names at the moment he cannot quite recall—who complained that Shakespeare's romances lack motivation and coherence, who called them moldy or meanly written, lame, vigorless, or absurd. It's not their wide gaps in time John objects to now, not their shallow characters or their knotty plots, not their strange mix of moods—comedy piled on tragedy like peppermint on licorice in the double-scoop ice cream his brother once dared him to eat. It's not even that those plays are cut of the same fabric from which myths and folktales come. It's that the particular myths they harken to are hoaxes, the tales they are bred from filled with baseless promises—or cruel lies.

It is requir'd You do awake your faith, commands Paulina in the final scene of *The Winter's Tale* as she restores the statue Hermione has been to her own dear life again. Once upon a time John had called that scene sublime. But tonight he cannot forget that Hermione's transformation from stone to flesh is not a real epiphany but only a cheap theatrical trick. Tonight he is appalled to realize that, like all the characters simpering through their happy tears onstage, he ever let himself forget the true costs of that moment: Paulina's husband devoured by a bear, Hermione and Leontes's son long dead, their daughter Perdita raised apart, and the witty and forthright Hermione so silenced after her awakening that she might as well still be made of marble.

Forget and forgive, Lord Cleomenes advises King Leontes, and soon Leontes is rewarded with a lovely daughter and a living wife. *Forget and forgive*, John broods in his lonely bed—as if forgiveness can mean anything if forgetting comes first, as if forgiveness matters more than understanding. But it's understanding that lends the comedies their happy endings. It's understanding that makes the tragedies so much more than sorry tales. It's understanding—not forgetting—that humans need and crave. It's understanding that John still strains for, even in this poor cell.

"I don't unnerstan." In his mind's ear he hears someone making that complaint. In his mind's lap, he feels her, too, perched like a sparrow on his thighs and knees as she leans towards the bright little book he holds in front of them. "The. Sun." She is straining to name the letters on the page, struggling to match those names to sounds, trying to make those sounds fit into words.

"Did. Not." Word by word she trudges across the page, serious as a spelunker entering a dark new cave, and when she reaches a word that makes no sense to her—*shine*, for example, with its feigning final *e*, she announces her confusion more as an affront than an admission. "I don't unnerstan."

"It. Was. Too. Wet. To play." She can't be more than four, and she is working so hard she is nearly shaking. "So. We. Sat. In the. House.

"All that. Cold, cold. Wet. Day." He remembers her pride when she deciphers the first page, her delighted, excited, breathless conviction that reading is the key to everything.

He'd believed that, too, he thinks now with a pang. He'd believed that words and stories and literature could teach people how to think and how to feel, that art could alter the world. He'd staked his life on that.

Reade him. That's what those saints John Heminge and Henry Condell wrote in the preface to their collection of William Shakespeare's plays, the Folio they published seven years after his death in their attempt to still time and keep the memory of their sweet friend and worthy colleague alive.

Reade him, they advised, *and againe, and againe. And if then you doe not like him, surely you are in some manifest danger, not to understand him.*

Reade him. That's what John has always urged his students— freshmen or graduate students alike. He tells them not to worry about the criticism, not to pay too much attention to what anyone else has said. Just read him for yourself, read him until you understand him.

And let him read you.

Though now he thinks it was all for naught, all that reading, all that care and work. Like Prospero, the magician and sometime Duke of Milan in Shakespeare's last great *Tempest*, he had dedicated his life to studying the liberal arts and bettering his mind. But look where it ended him—warehoused in some lonely cell with nothing to show for all his labor but defeat, regret, and yearning.

For years he'd tried to tease his students toward epiphanies, had striven to entice them with the delights of thinking and the promise of understanding, but tonight he wonders if even one of them was ever really affected by his efforts.

He'd placed his faith in literature and the liberal arts. But art is not potatoes. He'd known that long ago. Art cheats and mocks and misleads. It's the airiest of nothings, the basest of all lies. If it's Prospero's so potent art that lends him the magic he needs to rule his isle, trap his enemies, and make his daughter a queen, in the end it's that same art that Prospero must abjure simply to win his dukedom back again.

Closing his eyes, John listens as familiar voices come clamoring to speak his griefs. *Thou wouldst not think how ill all's here about my heart   Write sorrow on the bosom of the earth   I have of late—but wherefore I know not—lost all my mirth*

So much has been lost—not just mirth—but everything that matters. So much has been banished or forgot, so much ruined or misconstrued. *The jaws of darkness do devour it up   All's cheerless, dark, and deadly.   The best is past   Thou'lt come no more*

Sally said there was still time. But Sally is gone now, too.

Suddenly, he is sobbing. He is crying as if he has always been crying, crying as if he will never stop, crying for every loss he has ever known, for all the losses still to come. Sobs rip his chest, tears sting his cheeks. So much is wrong, so much is gone, and what little is left cannot piece out any comfort at all.

"Mistah Wilson, Mistah Wilson, wat's de matter?" A hand rests on his shoulder. He looks up through his tears at the bottom of a woman's face, her tawny neck and chin, her small dark nostrils. "Wat's wrong?" she asks. "Is dere anyt'ing you want?"

There are so many matters, so many wrongs, so many things he wants. It dizzies him to try to name them all. He wants his mother back, and wants his dear wife. He wants his daughter to return in time, wants her to uncurse him, to understand his point of view. He wants enough sleep, wants his speech written down in front of him, wants his audience to listen to him.

But suddenly he is accosted by the biggest wrong of all, the epiphany that reduces every other matter to dust:

It was right for his speech to be a failure.

It was right for his speech to be a failure, since what he had been defending was a lie.

ANOTHER DAY.

Or perhaps the same day, in this strange disjointed time, in which great swaths of his life seem to have never happened, while other moments keep returning like old friends. Or bad pennies. Or the *Twilight Zone* reruns Barb used to stare at on TV.

He's sitting in some anonymous green room, sitting in a leathern chair he swears he recognizes from some other where, watching out of a picture window as leaves swirl and fall, golden leaves that caper in the air like glowing garden sprites. He can watch those leaves forever, their twirl and loll. He'd forgotten—or had he never known?—how beautiful a falling leaf can be.

Sally comes to see him. Speaking of beauty. Sally, his bee holder. She comes sometimes, though never enough, and never now. Never when he needs her as much as he needs her in this very now.

Sometimes she stays away so long he forgets she has ever been, so that when she returns, he has to learn her all over again. Though other times when she's gone he can't forget her for a minute, and he keeps asking after her, asking and asking and asking when she will come again.

Her face is thin and worried when she comes, and her pain pains him. She hugs him, holds him, prates, and strokes his hand.

185

She says she misses him, claims that nothing's the same without him, that she thinks about him all the time. She tells him she's been working hard. She says her bees are thriving, promises she'll be able to spend more time with him soon, now that the hives are nearly winterized. It's been a good year, she tells him, she thinks she'll be able to keep the business, stay in their home. She tells him she's proud of him, says she knows this hasn't been easy, wishes there'd been any other way. She tells him he's been brave and selfless. She says she loves him.

Her eyes say she loves him, too, though her voice sounds tired and lorn, so weary it cracks his heart. He nearly wishes she did not love him, it seems to hurt her so.

Now and then, when she sees he is feeling talkative, she'll ask him about a play. Then she'll hold his hand and listen as he recites some lines or expounds on what he knows. Sometimes the plots confound him, and sometimes characters wander in from other plays, but often both he and she are surprised at how much he still has to say.

He has been ruminating on the romances mainly, or trying to, because even in this meager chamber there are so many interruptions to his work. A moaning crone. A dancing leaf. A lass come to mop the floor. He has been thinking about those beguiling romances—though he can't always recall their names—how they pretend that errors can be forgiven, that families can be reunited and kingdoms can be restored, how they try to claim that life is so rife with second chances that even people who were lost at sea or changed to stone can return to their homes and resume their loves unharmed.

Once he had argued that their lack of realism is in service of a higher truth, but now that he is two decades older than Shakespeare ever lived to be, now that he has seen what Shakespeare did not live to see, John regrets he ever defended those final plays. Because despite their glister and shimmer, despite the lilt of their poetry and the loveliness of their songs, in the end they take the coward's way out, valuing faith and forgetting more than growth and understanding.

But the tragedies feign, too. Or at least he suspects they do. With their blithe advice to go forth and have more talk of these sad things, with their implication that a man might understand his life before he leaves it, don't they, too, try to pretend there is more than dusty nothing waiting at the end?

"A story's only sad if it ends before things get happy again." He remembers someone saying that, a little grave-eyed girl. He remembers her climbing onto his lap, remembers her wiggling to get comfortable with a proprietorial ease that pleases him no end, remembers her solemn explanation, "It's like how if 'Little Red Riding Hood' had stopped after the wolf had aten Grandmother instead of waiting till the woodcutter chopped her out. You have to wait for the ending you like," she adds with stern conviction, "and then stop there."

He remembers feeling charmed and proud, remembers thinking how many happy endings the world must surely hold for a girl who understood the shape of stories so well. But she was wrong, John thinks, staring back into a bitter past. And he was wrong not to warn her, there and then. Because beyond every happy ending is another tragedy. And beyond the final tragedy is mere oblivion.

That woman is back. Not his beloved copesmate, but the other, wafting one. He is glad and sad and mad to see her, such a muddy stew of simple feelings, like red and blue and yellow crayons all blended into brown.

"Dad!" she announces gaily, as if that in itself were a good thing. She wears hempen breeches, a parti-colored jerkin, her hair looks tempest tossed.

"A piece of him," John agrees charily. But something stirs in the regions of his heart, not a spark exactly but the dull glower of long-banked coals. He's seen her before, he's sure of it, though she seems different now. She's changed, even if he can't say exactly how. He wonders why she has sought him out in this hollow cell.

"Why are you here?" he wonders aloud.

"I wanted to see you, Dad," she says as she sits down. "I wanted to see how you're doing, maybe give it another chance." But her voice sounds too hale, the laugh she ends her wants with seems oddly culpable. He is not at all sure he should place his trust in her.

Out on the lawn, a man appears with a wheelbarrow and a rake. Planting the barrow by the wall, he commences to comb the turf for golden leaves.

"I've been thinking," John says at length. "About . . . green worlds."

"What?"

"Green worlds. Where characters go," he continues, his voice gaining a lecturer's timbre despite how he stumbles among his words, "to be, transformed. Topsy . . . turvy places. Like mazes, carnivals. Beyond the hardened . . . hierarchies, city or . . . court. Outside of time. They're where the greatest change . . . occurs, not in . . . cremental, but . . . almost instant. As if, confusion is all . . . it, takes."

"Oh, right," she answers swiftly. "I remember. Green worlds—you talked about them last time, too."

"Green worlds," he agrees, "and not just . . . the comedies or . . . romances. *Lear*, too, I . . . think, the . . . heath," John offers as the barrow man gathers a golden pile. "Maybe Juliet's . . . orchard. Even Falstaff's . . . green fields. But. It's all a . . . jokes—a hoax, I mean. A lie." He gives a harsh, hard sigh.

"Green worlds don't exist," he says, shifting his gaze from the raker to focus on his daughter.

"Well, sure," she laughs, "They're made-up stories."

"A hoax," he answers sternly. Speaking rapidly as if he were determined to finish his thought before it vanishes, he continues, "Stories, art, poetry, even. The . . . plays. You don't see, it . . . last. I mean, don't see . . . the last, of it. The change comes. And the play ends. We never see. How, it plays . . . out. Freya was right," he ends bitterly, "It was all a dead. White man's . . . game."

"A game?" she echoes with a sudden keen interest, and though her question is equivocal, it seems to ease his mood a little.

"I've forgotten," he replies, "where you went, to . . . college."

"I didn't go." She speaks quickly, and suddenly her tone seems nervous, even needy. "I mean, I haven't yet. But I've been trying, these last few months. I've been working really hard at it. I got accepted and everything. I was supposed to start in January."

She pauses, watching out the window as the man crams his glowing piles into a black plastic bag like a billowing shroud. "But two weeks ago I got the financial aid package, and now I don't see how I can possibly do it." When she continues, her voice is brittle. "I've crunched the numbers a million times, and there's just no way I could go without ending up at least a hundred thousand dollars in debt.

"I could swing some debt, of course. But one hundred thousand dollars just sounds insane. I've looked into scholarships," she plows on, "but there's not a lot out there for game designers—and especially not returning students who barely even managed to graduate high school. I found one, and I've been working on it, but frankly, I don't see how I could possibly win it. They want you to come up with an entire proposal for a game, an outline that covers everything from the story and artwork to gameplay and mechanics and technical interfaces."

She sags her head wearily from side to side. "It's a huge, huge project, like building a whole house or writing a novel or a symphony or something. And I'm just a beginner. I don't know nearly enough yet to design an entire game. It's like you need to have a degree already before you'd even have a chance."

She takes a quick breath, holds it for a second, and then blurts in a rush, "Dad, before, when I was here the last time, you said there was some money set aside for my education, and I've been thinking. I have no idea how much there is—or if it even still exists—but I was wondering, maybe, I mean, do you think maybe I could use some of it? I wouldn't ask," she pushes on, "but I really don't see how I can go to college without it. There's just no way. I found out online that some people have been working on their designs for that scholarship for years."

"That education . . . money's for my . . . daughter. To educate my, daughter," he says, frowning as the man with the barrow wheels his load offstage.

"I know," she nods happily. "That's me, Dad—I'm your daughter. It would be just so great if I could use some of it."

"Daughter." He gives her a long steady look, and the recognition in his expression seems firm and warm. "If there be truth in sight, you are my daughter."

"Yes, yes—that's right. I'm your daughter."

"Sweet daughter," he muses out the window where a few final leaves are drifting from the tree like lost chances, "short daughter . . . dow'rless . . . peddler's daughter . . . 'I have a daughter that I love passing well— '"

"Passing?" she gives an awkward little laugh.

"Exceedingly," he explains promptly. "Polonius means, he loves . . . her . . . exceedingly. Though with that . . . rat, it's always hard to tell. Daughter," he continues contentedly, as if inviting other allusions to come. "Gentle . . . fair . . . sole . . . 'I have another daughter, Who I am sure is kind and comfortable.'"

"That's me," the woman beside him answers, her voice fond and teasing. "That's me, Dad—your sole, fair, kind and comfortable daughter."

"Kind and comfortable?" His eyes widen and he shakes his head violently. "You?"

"You bet," she laughs. "Your kind and comfortable daughter."

"Kind and comfortable?" he glares at her. "Never. Not . . . you."

"Dad—" she begins.

"Unnatural hag," he announces indignantly, "is what, that . . . daughter, is. She'll die," he continues fiercely. "Before she ever . . . gets a penny. Kind and comfortable," he scoffs. "That's the daughter, who . . . cursed . . . she's, the one, who . . . ruined everything."

"I was raped." She speaks softly, but something strong has entered her voice, not anger, not anguish, but something clear and unflinching. "That time in London, when I didn't come back to the hotel? I was raped."

When he does not respond, she goes on, "You thought I was being defiant when I wouldn't tell you more about where I'd been, but I was so scared and ashamed. It was all so confusing that for a long time I wasn't even sure myself exactly what happened. For years I couldn't bring myself to talk—or even really think—about it, partly because I believed it was all my fault, and partly because I was trying to pretend it didn't matter."

She turns to look him full in the face. "They were college boys, I think—from Belgium or Poland or somewhere. I met them in Trafalgar Square, and they took me to a pub. After the pub, we ended up in some kind of hostel, or maybe a dorm room. I should have left, but I could hardly walk by that point, and I had no idea where I was.

"I didn't like what was happening, how they kissed me, and . . . passed me around. But I was such a kid. I was too dumb and drunk and embarrassed and scared to escape. Besides, I was so dizzy I couldn't even keep my eyes open, and I had no idea where I was, or how to get back to the hotel."

She pauses to look to him. "Do you understand what I'm telling you?"

For an interminable time he does not appear to have heard her question, and when he finally answers, "Enough," his voice is so harsh and ragged that at first it seems he's commanding her to stop talking. But when she glances over at him, his face is drawn, his expression ravaged.

"It was horrible," she continues. "I was—is there a word for beyond embarrassed, or ashamed? I felt responsible for what happened to you, too, with your speech and all. I felt so awful, Dad." Her voice is thin and ragged. "I thought I'd ruined everything."

"Calchas," he croaks, shutting his eyes, "traitor, I never . . . Woeful, Cressida."

She waits for him to open his eyes or maybe to say something more, and when he doesn't, she shakes her head as if to clear it of his gibberish, "After I got back to California my period was way late. When I finally realized I was pregnant, I called you, and talked to Freya. I waited for you to call back," She breaks off to take a shuddering breath, but her words sound strong when she continues. "But you never did. And before I could gather up my courage to call you again, I had a miscarriage."

He sits with his eyes closed, still as stone, while his daughter says, "For a long time after that, it seemed easier for us to just go our separate ways, though I never stopped hoping that someday we'd find a way to get past all that crap, to forgive each other, and start again." Her words fade into her thoughts, and when she finally speaks again, her voice has a stabbing edge. "But that was another stupid fantasy. You're right, Dad. It's all a hoax. That story—it's nothing but a lie."

"Go," he whispers behind shut eyelids. "Leave," he says more urgently. "It's too, late. Now. Get you . . . gone."

For a moment she hesitates, looking down into his closed face, even reaching a tentative hand toward his shoulder. But before her fingers can make contact with the fabric of his shirt, he barks, "Who is't that hinders you?"

Randi is trembling by the time she bursts through the front doors, so sickened and shaken and ashamed, it is as if she'd never left that shoddy London room at all, as if she was still as numb and dumb and naked as ever, still unable to even try to stop those leering boys.

She yearns to have a cigarette before she starts the long drive home, but she can't bear the thought of running into anyone in the smoking area. She fears that Tony, with his dorky jokes and corny encouragement, might be the worst. Instead, she races down the white sidewalk, buzzes herself through the locked gate, then stumbles across the asphalt to her car.

When she reaches it, she unlocks the door and throws herself into the driver's seat. Leaning forward, she rests her forehead on the steering wheel, tries to get the seethe to settle in her chest. She feels raw—both skin and soul—suddenly utterly overcome by who she is and what she's hoped for.

She should have never told him about London. She hadn't meant to, though there had been a time when she'd longed for him to know her side of that gruesome tale. She'd hoped that someday they could sort out the causes and the consequences of that trip together. She had even imagined they might come to an understanding, that they might forgive each other at last, safe inside the mobius of their mutual love.

But she'd given up trying to fix the past—or at least she thought she had. She'd come today in hopes of finding a future instead. Her forehead still pressed against the steering wheel, she sighs and shakes her head. She should never have asked him for that money.

She'd known from the beginning it was wrong. But she had been so desperate to go to ArtTech, and that education fund had been her last real chance.

Two weeks ago, after she finished reading the message from ArtTech outlining her financial obligations, she'd stared at the smoke undulating from her cigarette, and it had been like watching her entire destiny fade with it into the empty air. Ever since then she'd felt the familiar tug of numbness, that yearning to return to being careful, small and dull. It was that feeling she was trying to fight when she resolved to ask her father for help.

"He misses you," Sally said when she'd called again last week.

"How do you know?" Randi asked.

"The stories he keeps telling about when you were little, for one thing."

"I'm not little anymore." She had been taking extra shifts to save more money, and then racing home to work on her scholarship. She'd decided to design a game based on the world she'd described in her admissions application, and for the first few weeks it had been more lark than work as she dreamed up characters and imagined features and developed narrative elements. But the longer she spent on it, the more gaps and contradictions began to pop up, and every idea she found to try to fix them seemed immature and uninspired, every workaround she devised only revealed further problems, only highlighted how little she really knew.

The deadline was still ten weeks away, but it was already obvious she couldn't possibly win. It was like trying to build a castle out of jello, like trying to paint the wind or sail across an ocean on a raft made of flower petals. Every night it took more courage for her to get back to work on it, and she knew the night was coming when she wouldn't be able to force herself to work on it at all.

"Can I tell you a story?" Sally asked suddenly.

"A story?" she echoed cautiously. On her computer screen, the list of game elements she still needed to design seemed like an enumeration of all her failures yet to come.

"Have you ever heard of the Freedom Riders?"

A vague memory from high school history class stirred in Randi's head. She said, "I guess so, but I don't really—"

"Back in the early sixties, those busloads of students who rode through the South, trying to enforce desegregation. I was one of them."

"Wow," Randi said politely, waiting for the gap that would let her end the conversation and try to get back to work.

"It was quite a trip," Sally answered drily, "much harder than I'd ever imagined anything could be before I got on that bus. We were cursed, threatened, spat on. We'd pledged to practice nonviolence, so we couldn't react to any of the threats or even the abuse. I never actually got beaten, but most of the men did. We ended up in the prison, in Jackson. They gave me a body cavity search it took years to recover from." Although Sally's voice was even and calm, her words jolted Randi's gaze from the screen.

"But that's a different story for another time," Sally ended lightly.

In the pause that followed, there were things Randi wanted to ask Sally, things she suddenly felt like saying, but they came crowding in all at once and, before she could offer anything, Sally went on, "When I told my parents I was going south that summer, they said if I was going to be a part of that, I could no longer be their daughter. I was an only child, so you can imagine it was quite an ultimatum.

"My parents were good people in many ways. I understand that now. They were limited, and uneducated, and shaped by their culture, but they were also hardworking and determined, and—" Sally gave an ironic laugh "—committed to their values. But I was so disturbed by their racism and by how they were trying to rule my life that I couldn't see anything else. I told them if that was the way they wanted it, it was fine with me. I was twenty, and before I left I said that I would make sure they always had my address, but until they were willing to accept me for who I was, I wouldn't have anything more to do with them.

"So for the next fifteen years, every time I moved I sent them a postcard with my new address on it. And that whole time I never heard a single word from them. I kept telling myself I was doing the right thing, that we had irreconcilable differences, that it was better for all three of us if we didn't see each other until they realized how wrong they'd been."

Despite what Sally was saying, there was something almost soothing about her quiet voice, the way her story seemed to turn that painful past into a place as tidy and precise as a landscape seen from a plane. "But one day," she continued, "almost on a whim, I decided we weren't any of us getting any younger, so I called them. I used the same number we'd had when I was a kid. A distant cousin of my mom's answered. She said she'd been trying to find me. My folks had been in a car wreck the week before, and both of them were dead."

Randi made an inadvertent gasp. She was groping for something to say when Sally continued, "I have to admit there were times when I might have said it would be for the best, for my parents to just pass on without our ever having to see each other again, much less having to try to work things out. And—who knows?—even if I'd made that call before they died, it might still have been a losing battle. There are parts of ourselves I believe we should never give up—not even for love."

Sally gave a soft little laugh. "I had to learn that lesson the hard way, too. I think my first husband and I stayed together much longer than we should have because I was so traumatized by losing my parents like that.

"Though it worked out in the end, didn't it?" she added, the sheen returning to her voice, "since I can't imagine your father and I would have been ready for each other a whole lot sooner."

And so, prodded by Sally's story and driven by her own rash needs, she attempted one last visit to her father. "Third time's the charm," she'd quipped to Mink that morning as she was starting out, and she'd been grateful when he desisted from observing what he'd warned her of before—that one definition of insanity was doing the same thing over and over and expecting different results.

Well, she did get different results, she thinks grimly, as she straightens up and jams her key into the ignition. This time, she not only lost her father but her chance at ArtTech, too.

"Who is 't that hinders you?" is what her father asked when he was goading her to leave. As she pulls out of the parking lot, she is much too morose to entertain that question. But later, on the freeway, halfway through the long drone home, after she has finished sobbing and swearing, and her eyes itch from crying and her throat aches from screaming and her palms sting from slapping the steering wheel, an answer comes to her anyway, an answer with an emotional twang like a country-western song, a line whose provenance she cannot trace although its meaning suddenly seems excruciatingly exact: *A foolish heart, that I leave here behind.*

Something bad has happened, something has gone badly wrong. Something that hurts and irks in equal measure.

Despite his aching hip, John circles his room like a wrathful dragon, stalks his same cramped round past window, dresser, door, and door. His daughter has come. And gone. Again. At first he'd thought she'd come to see him, that she wanted to be his friend, that things might still come right between them. But instead she'd come bearing tales it tortured him to hear, and when he tried to let her know how wronged she'd been—like woeful Cressida passed from man to man among the merry Greeks while her traitorous blundering father seals poor Cressid's doom—she'd scorned his concern, raced off, left him to anguish still in this damn'd green gaol.

Window, dresser, door, and door. His hip hurts hard. He limps and moans. She's gone forever. She'll come no more. Traitors all. There is a photo on the dresser. He notes it in passing—Sally smiling at the camera from the orchestra of an ancient theater, John standing beside her, a smile pasted on his face, too. The more fool he, he snarls in his mind as he marches past.

There is a book on the dresser. It catches his eye on his next round. He's noticed it before, though he can't say where or why. It is a gaudy thing, he sees when he pauses to glare at it. With its gold lettering and its cover blazoned with the Chandos portrait, it's the kind of volume he has always scorned for the way it implies the plays must be pranked up to prove their worth. He wonders how it got there, that foolish garish tome, marvels at what strange route it must have taken to reach him in that bootless, bookless room.

The image of a woman wafts into his thoughts. An eager, drifting woman. Not Sally, but someone else. He sees her brimming smile as she urges the book on him. Even now, the afterimage of that smile lingers in his mind like the grin of the Cheshire Cat in a story he once read to some young child. He sees her rumpled hair, too, and hears her voice—soft, gentle and low.

Remembering, he is suffused with a pleasure satisfying as the taste of salt on steak. He longs to have that woman with him now, though along with his longing, he feels a grating of indignation. It is not fair for her to have cursed him as she did, not fair for her to have left and not taken him.

He wonders who could have raised such a thoughtless, thankless child.

Still clutching the foppish book, he stumbles back to the small haven of his chair, sinks dully down. Taking up a chunk of pages, he lets them spill across his fingertips, catching words and random phrases *bastard   sack   chafed   incarnadine   nothing either good or bad   My mistress with a monster   fools into a circle*

Words, he thinks contemptuously as they pour past—*words, words, words   empty words   foul words   mere words* He gave his life to them, and what did they give him back? He should have sold used cars instead.

alms for oblivion   how I may compare This prison where I live unto the world   there rust, and let me die

I thought the King had more affected the Duke of Albany than Cornwall. When those words snag his eyes, John lets the page fall flat, the seeming-simple line that begins *King Lear* lying quietly beneath his gaze.

King Lear—what the First Quarto calls the *historie* and the Folio calls the *tragedie*. Looking down at that pristine page, John feels a sudden pang of longing for his teaching copy. Its spine long broken, its pages yellowed and folded, it was exactly the sort of thing the clay-brained clotpole he hired to help him pack his office wanted to throw out. Idiot kid, he hadn't conceived the treasure that book had been, each scene—and nearly every line—fortified with half a century's worth of notes, some penciled in the careful hand of John's earliest days as a teacher, others, much later, dashed off in ink, questions and observations and concordances, notes where the editor's choices diverged from his own—the Quarto's *they cannot touch me for coining* instead of the Folio's *they cannot touch me for crying*, the Folio's *consumption* in the sulfurous pit of hell instead of the Quarto's *consummation*—his own extra glosses to help explain to his students the difference between a natural and an artificial fool, or describe the Elizabethan notion of fortune's wheel, or the divine right of kings.

For a stinging moment, the thought of that lost book hurts him nearly past endurance. But Kent's observation about the King's affections awaits an answer, and John can hardly help but read Gloucester's gossipy reply: *It did always seem so to us; but now in the division of the kingdom, it appears not which of the Dukes he values most.*

The last time he'd tried to read Shakespeare, some jester had played a joke on him, substituting a foul copy or a trick version for the true text of the play. Since then he's been wary of getting cozened like that again. But now the lines in his lap seem blessedly clear. When plainspoken Kent tells Gloucester he cannot conceive him, and the weak old lecher Gloucester quips that his bastard son's mother could, John chuckles at the joke even as he cringes for Edmund's feelings and hopes he hasn't overheard his father's crude boast.

Attend the lords of France and Burgundy, announces Lear as he and his retinue sweep into the scene. And already King Lear is entering his council room, already announcing, *Mean time we shall express our darker purpose.* Already a welcome thrill is arcing through John's brain, so that instead of succumbing to his grim new insights about the limitations of language and the meagerness of theater, instead of being frustrated by how little scholarship and background knowledge he has left to bring to that opening scene, he is swept along by the story itself.

Which of you shall we say doth love us most the vain old king demands, and John watches in disgust as Goneril and Regan flatter and grovel, watches in fear as forthright Cordelia refuses to coddle the dragon even in his wrath. *So young, my lord, and true.*

Better thou Hadst not been born than not t' have pleas'd me better. With its odd mix of domesticity and histrionics, *King Lear* has never been John's favorite of the great tragedies. But he finishes the first scene grateful to have entered Lear's world and left his own behind. As the words wrap around him and the plot pulls him on, it's as if Lear's troubles were a balm for all his own.

Thy dow'rless daughter, King, thrown to my chance, Is queen of us, of ours, and our fair France.   *This is the excellent foppery of the world*   *Not so young, sir, to love a woman for singing, nor so old to dote on her for any thing* In addition to his relief at the asylum he's found inside the play, he finds himself amazed at the excruciating beauty of it. Line after line strikes him, so fresh and astonishing he wonders if he ever actually read *King Lear* before.

He finds so much that touches him, so much he yearns to share. His pang when Lear cries, *Who is it that can tell me who I am?* His spark of epiphany when the Fool replies, *Lear's shadow.* His wince of recognition and regret when the Fool advises his royal master, *Thou shouldst not have been old till thou hadst been wise*—so many moments John wishes he could teach or discuss with Sally or tell the world about.

But there are also things he does not understand, such as the extent of his own anguish when, in the midst of the Fool's riddling about crabs and noses, Lear interrupts his prattle to lament, *I did her wrong.*

I did her wrong. Such a simple declaration. Four words, four syllables, two easy iambs—and yet that little sentence comes near to skewering him, such a painful puzzle he gladly lets his thoughts veer elsewhere.

Of course he's never seen a perfect production of *King Lear*, though the Eyre performance at the National Theatre came close, with Ian Holm capturing the tenderness of the old tyrant, if not quite all his majesty. He'd seen the Peter Brook production, too, that time with Nancy in Stratford-upon-Avon. It had been hailed as a masterpiece, though Nancy was bored by its glacial pace, and John found it too brutal, too austere—impossible to believe a Lear so cold could ever have deserved the love that Cordelia, Kent, Edgar, Gloucester, and the Fool professed for him. Maybe Richard Burbage, the actor for whom Shakespeare wrote Lear's role, managed to do the old king justice, though John had long agreed with all those other critics, from Lamb to Bloom, who claim that King Lear's character is too vast for any stage, that only in the human imagination can his plight and personality have ample room.

The art of our necessities is strange, And can make vild things precious. Looking up from the page, John gazes dispassionately at the few new-fallen leaves spotting the darkening lawn while thunder cracks, and Lear's storm drenches the heath. When he looks down again, the Fool is singing *heigh-ho, the wind and the rain*, and prophesying confusion. Then John is back inside Gloucester's castle, watching in dread while Gloucester confides his loyalty to King Lear to his treacherous son, Edmund. And anon John is back in the storm as Kent points to the pitiful hovel and pleads, *Good my lord, enter here.*

When loyal Edgar, disguised as lunatic Poor Tom, bursts out of the hovel to writhe in the mud at King Lear's feet, John stands in Lear's stead, gazing down upon that poor, bare, forked animal and asking the question that drives the play, *Is man no more than this?* He feels those words shudder through him, the bleak summation of his entire life, his futile hopes, his failed quest, feels the cold downpour on his bare head, the chill drops fingering their way beneath his sodden cloak, the wind-driven rain blast his face like sand, feels the outrage of despair and the universe's vast indifference, and then, a moment later, he feels a sweep of gratitude which can only be called love when Gloucester enters with his torch to guide them to a dry hovel hard by, urging, *No words, no words, hush.*

Hang him instantly, Regan is suggesting of Gloucester while her sister Goneril hisses, *Pluck out his eyes*, when some ignorant wench pokes her head into John's room to announce that it is movie and popcorn time. But John growls and swats the air, and even before the interloper has loped on down the hall, he is back in Gloucester's castle, listening in horror as Regan and Cornwall taunt their old host, watching aghast as Regan, the daughter Lear had so recently called kind and comfortable, curses Gloucester and plucks his white beard. When Cornwall sets his foot upon the first of Gloucester's eyes, John gasps out loud. A second later he knows a thrill of relief to hear Cornwall's servant cry, *Hold your hand, my lord!*

Despite the hope that quickens at the thought that Gloucester might still be spared, John reads on in helpless horror as kind and comfortable Regan slays that nameless peasant and wounded Cornwall pries out Gloucester's other eye, reads on, appalled, as kind and comfortable Regan orders the newly-blinded Gloucester thrust out at gates to smell his way to Dover.

It is when Gloucester's loyal son, Edgar, still disguised as a mad Bedlam beggar, claims, *The lowest and most dejected thing of fortune Stands still in esperance*, that John realizes he cannot remember whether Edgar is ever reunited with his father, cannot even recall if Gloucester lives or dies. Yanking his gaze from the page, he clutches the book in both bent fists and strains against the mean bonds of his mind, struggling to recall any hint or inkling that would help restore his memory of Gloucester's fate. Or Lear's fate, for that matter, or Edgar's or Cordelia's—for suddenly he realizes he cannot recall any aspect of the ending of the play.

He has studied Shakespeare's work for the length of Shakespeare's lifetime, but he has forgotten how *King Lear* ends. Clinging to the book as if it alone can save him, he strives with all his power to recall the climax of the play. He suspects that things do not work out well— *King Lear* is a tragedy, after all—but strain as he might, he cannot recall what happens next. Desperately, he scans the room, seeking any refuge. But it seems he is on the deck of a tilting ship as it lifts and lists and plunges into dark water.

"Oh, gods," he moans, burying his eyes and forehead in his cupped palms, grinding his thumbs into his temples. "Please," he whispers, nearly whimpering, though whether he is pleading for himself and his tattered memory or for the fates of Lear and Gloucester, Edgar and Cordelia, he cannot say. He only knows that something huge is at stake, as if the outcome of everything that ever mattered rests upon the conclusion of that play. Suddenly, it seems that even more momentous than the fact that after fifty years he has forgotten how *King Lear* ends, is that—however it ends—that ending means everything.

Consumed by his need to follow wherever the play leads, he keeps reading, reads with deep foreboding and bated hope, and sometimes he is Gloucester, blood dripping from the empty sockets of his lost eyes as he shuffles toward the cliff's edge in his mind. Sometimes he is Edgar, promising that the worst is yet to come as he leads his father toward that false abyss. And sometimes he is the King himself, railing against lechery, wiping the scent of mortality from his hand, counseling the ruined Gloucester to patience: *When we are born, we cry that we are come To this great stage of fools.*

He can't remember how the story ends, but after fifty years of studying it, Elizabethan English is his native tongue. Not once does he have to pause to unravel the syntax of a line or consult the glosses for a word's meaning, not once does he even feel the absence of his own marginal notes. Only the story is new, and he reads it like a smug bridegroom, terrified and in love, hoping for the best with his whole untutored heart. No longer critical, no longer mercenary, he reads with no more motive than his thirst to be immersed in the language, no more desire than his hunger to discover what happens next, no other wish but that the characters he cares about so deeply will win the ends that they deserve, no need but that the play will somehow help him to make sense of the folly and conundrum of his own precious life.

When Lear and Cordelia are finally reunited, John knows such an upwelling of gratitude it is as if all sorrows that ever he has felt have been redeemed. When Lear confesses to his daughter, *I am a very foolish fond old man,*

> *Fourscore and upward, not an hour more nor less;*
> *And to deal plainly,*
> *I fear I am not in my perfect mind,*

John wonders if he might drown in the pity and joy he feels. And when Lear relies on the prick of a pin and the wetness of Cordelia's tears to assure himself he is neither dead nor dreaming, John is moved nearly to tears himself to think that pain and sorrow are the clues Lear uses to prove that he still lives.

But a few lines later, when Lear tells Cordelia, *Pray you now forget, and forgive: I am old and foolish*, John stops reading as if he, himself, has just been pricked awake.

Or mortally stabbed.

Forget, and forgive. He is outraged to find that lie lurking in *King Lear*, too. *Forget, and forgive*—not only in the romances but in fierce and seething *Lear*? *Forget, and forgive*, like some fatuous religious tract or foolish fairy tale. As if forgetting were a virtue, and forgiveness were more important than understanding.

Forget and forgive. He'd known it was there. Hadn't he? Surely he had known that vapid sentiment tainted *King Lear*, too.

Had he forgotten?

Or perhaps he'd known but had not understood. Maybe he hadn't recognized what was there beneath his very nose. Has his whole life been like that? he marvels and mourns. Has he been so busy studying that he missed the lie of everything?

The thought of a daughter floods him. Girl, infant, woman—his memories of her flicker like flames in wind. But though he cannot make her face resolve into a single image, he is suddenly stricken with both her being and her absence. He feels the lack of her like an ache in a lost limb. It seems that things have not ended well between them, although for all his life, he remembers not how or why.

But how or why is nothing to his urgent need to reach her, to find her and try to save her—now, before it is too late. "Run, run, O, run!" he groans, struggling to his feet. But wavering upright beside his chair, he is suddenly flummoxed by how to start. Beyond the window glass, another golden leaf glides down as if emergencies did not exist, as if life itself would last forever even as it drops away. Still clutched

205

in panic, John scrutinizes the placid grass, straining to calculate all the arcane phone numbers and addresses he'd need to reach her.

It's when he begins to consider how he might apologize or make amends for things he cannot recall that he sees how hopeless his situation is. He feels the prick and wetness of his failure, feels the awful inescapable emptiness of what is. "I did her wrong," he says, his voice breaking out unfettered in the still green room.

I did her wrong. Though what wrong those words are meant to name he cannot tell, still saying them seems to offer him some small ease, as if a noose were loosened or a burden lightened, as if a tender hand were stroking his old brow.

Soothed and newly broken, he sinks back into his chair, back into *Lear.* And still the words leap up to meet him, still they pull him in and sweep him on, past Regan and Goneril's machinations for Edmund's twisted affections, past Edmund's icy calculations about which sister he should take, to the very moment where Edmund arrives in post-battle triumph to order his officers to take the captives Lear and Cordelia away to prison.

But shaking off the officers, Lear ignores Gloucester's evil son. Speaking only to Cordelia, he vows, *When thou dost ask me blessing, I'll kneel down*

> *And ask of thee forgiveness. So we'll live,*
> *And pray, and sing, and tell old tales, and laugh*
> *At gilded butterflies*

"'And take upon 's the mystery of things,'" John whispers, rapt and ravaged. Lifting his eyes from the page, he gazes out at the autumnal world while the rest of Lear's line sounds in his mind like a celestial song, *As if we were God's spies*

He has forgotten the ending of the play, but he has not forgotten how to hope. Despite his years of scholarly reading and critical training, despite his own rejaundiced heart, still esperance pops up unbidden, irrepressible as the few fool-hearty dandelions that dot the leaf-strewn turf beyond the windowpane. So on he reads, tugged along by hope as Edmund's treachery is exposed and Edgar arrives to duel his heinous brother.

When the Gentleman enters with a bloody knife to announce, *O, she's dead!* John's first thought is that Cordelia has been slain, and he wonders how any father could endure such loss. A moment later, when he learns that the knife came from the heart of Goneril instead, he still dares hope that Cordelia and her father will be spared.

His waxing optimism that Edmund may do some good despite of his own nature matched with an ever-thickening dread when Edmund confesses his plan to have Cordelia hanged and lay the blame on her own despair that she foredid herself, John turns the page. But when Lear comes howling back from prison with Cordelia flopping like a rag doll in his arms, anguish blankets everything again.

O, you are men of stones! Lear accuses the stricken spectators when they fail to howl along with him. Bending over his daughter's body, he mourns, *She's gone for ever!* and, *She's dead as earth.* The final scene of *The Winter's Tale* flickers through John's mind, the stone statue of Leontes's long-dead wife awaking, the human woman descending from her pedestal to greet her daughter, forgive her husband, take up her mortal life once more. For a moment John hopes for a similar ending now, especially when the feather in Lear's trembling hand seems to show that Cordelia lives. *If it be so, It is a chance which does redeem all sorrows That ever I have felt.*

But instead, all chances are extinguished and every sorrow confirmed. Instead, Cordelia is gone forever, and the only crumb of comfort left anywhere is either the illusion created by the return of King Lear's madness, or the promise of an afterlife that only Lear can glimpse when he cries, *Look on her! Look her lips, Look there, look there!*

But before Lear can say what it is he sees, his fierce old heart has stopped, and suddenly John is alone once more—an old man weeping over the heap of ink and paper in his bony lap as he whispers the play's last lines along with Edgar.

"'The weight of this sad time we must obey,
Speak what we feel, not what we have to say:
The oldest hath borne most; we that are young
Shall never see so much, nor live so long.'"

Then, nothing.

Nothing but the stillness of his green room and the *I am* of his still-beating heart. Nothing but the small stir of his next breath and the monotonous leaking of his scalding tears—such a meager trickle compared to that torrential waste and loss and woe.

But such excruciating beauty, even so. He'd forgotten how much beauty, if he'd ever really known, beauty to flay his soul, beauty to leave him open and emptied and strangely whole, older but not the oldest, wiser only in that he recognizes he can never be wise enough. And so he sits, gutted and stunned and trying to understand, until a brisk stout lass who claims her name is Matty comes to lead him off to dinner.

In the dining room, the rabble shovels pork chops as if Cordelia were living still. The fulsome scents affront him, but he strives to bear free and patient thoughts, suffers himself to be settled at a table. The food they set before him is carrion and hay, but he eats it anyway.

He wonders what Lear sees—or thinks he sees—in that moment before he dies, wonders if it's an intimation of some true heaven or merely one last deception of the poor king's broken mind. He wonders if a true insight can come from a delusion, wonders if anything can be called an epiphany if it does not outlive the moment of its conception. Then he wonders if true epiphanies occur in any other way.

Back in his bedchamber, he wonders on. He knows he should

have answers to all these wonders, dimly suspects that he has studied and argued and opined on *Lear* for years. And yet all the skill he has remembers none of what he's read or what he's said, and he knows enough by now to understand that even the truth will never make all things plain.

"John," a woman calls from the doorway of his cell, "They're gonna have some music in the rec room before bedtime, Mrs. Wasson on the piano, for a little sing-along. You wanna come?"

"I'm busy," he snaps. "I've work to do. I'm running out of time."

"You sure? It would be good for you to socialize some more."

But he growls and waves the meddlesome wench away.

"Okay, then," she sighs as she moves on down the hall. "No singing for you."

He remembers singing.

He remembers trying to transmute a handful of lines into a tune for the sake of the infant screaming in his arms, a creature so tormented with gas or colic or existential despair that her face looks bee-stung and her little body arches and stiffens as she cries.

He has never sung for another person before. He knows he has a magnificent speaking voice. People tell him he reads beautifully. He can command the attention of a lecture hall full of freshmen with his voice alone. And yet his singing voice is surprisingly feeble. "Fear no more the heat o' th' sun," he begins in a croak, borrowing the words from Shakespeare's early romance *Cymbeline*.

"Nor the furious winter's rages." Groping for notes he is not sure he can find, he tries to turn the dirge King Cymbeline's rustic sons sing over the inert body of the youth they later discover to be their living sister into a lullaby:

"Thou thy worldly task hast done,
Home art gone, and ta'en thy wages."

Because Shakespeare's tune has not survived the centuries, John has had to cobble one of his own. He feels so uncertain at first—even at midnight, even in his own living room—it is as if he fears his brand-new daughter will interrupt her sobbing to criticize his song. But he is desperate for silence, desperate for sleep, desperate to make her crying quit, and so he persists, and slowly his voice grows more confident, slowly the melody becomes clearer as the hour wears on.

"Golden lads and girls all must, As chimney-sweepers, come to dust," he sings, taking pleasure in recalling that dandelions were called *golden lads* in Shakespeare's time, that dandelions gone to seed were known as *chimney sweepers*, savoring those homey proofs that whatever Will Shakespeare became, in some part of his great heart he was always a country lad.

"All lovers young, all lovers must Consign to thee and come to dust." They are the words of a lament and not a lullaby, and John feels a nibble of guilt or even superstition to be singing them to one so newly come to this great stage of fools. But somehow it seems right, too, to be sharing with that screaming barne both the beauty and the tragedy of the world she's been thrust into, as though he were warning her and promising her, even as he tries to shush her.

And gradually, a different quality seems to enter her wailing. It is as if her attention were being divided, as if she were listening even as she cries. Slowly the space between her sobs grows longer until finally, with one last deep shuddering exhalation, her eyes sag shut, and she is asleep. *Fear no more*

Pacing that tired square of floor, he'd been desperate to hush her, desperate to get her into her crib so that he can turn to his nightcap, his book and bed. But now, alongside his relief that she is finally sleeping, he wishes his success hadn't made him obsolete. He is oddly reluctant to return to the rest of his life: a drink, a book, a sleep—and then what? Gazing into her soft face, he believes that all his sorrows—both past and yet to come—can never be as full as that moment's joy.

Sitting in his dimming cell, he wonders where she is now, that infant so fresh from her coming hither. As the watch on his wrist ticks away forever, he wishes she were with him still, wishes he could retrace one single strand of time from the mingled yarn that is his life back to that long-ago midnight, and so recover that blossom he'd once loved with the whole of his newborn heart.

A woman enters. A dolorous moaning woman, who interrupts his reverie with such groans that she might be Ophelia when her wits have fled, or even Cassandra bewailing the disasters she alone can foresee, though when John turns to look at her, he finds no Trojan princess or young sweet maid, but a grandam, her gray hair bunned in some old-world way, who clutches a picture frame to her breast as if it were an icon or a prayer book.

"Aroint thee, witch," John snarls as is his wont whenever some wretch or knave invades his chamber. "Go shake your ears." But she ignores him. Keening a lament in some language that is Greek to him, she lowers herself into the empty chair that sits beside his own.

"Shog off," he snaps, and, "Hag-seed, hence." But when he darts his glare at her, he sees her wrinkled face is wet with tears, and it strikes him she may be lamenting for him, too, mourning his very griefs in her unknown human tongue.

"Hush," John whispers, borrowing the same soft sound that Gloucester uses to sooth the thunder-crazed King Lear. "Hush," he says again, and "hush," letting the little syllable balm his sorrows, too. *Hush.*

Reaching across the gap between their chairs, he covers her hand with his, keeps vigil while she wauls, sits beside her as her faithful guardant as the day's last light melts into night and the room fills up with living shadows and absent shades. Gradually, her weeping ceases. Slowly her prattle fades into a silence more tuneful than any song.

Perhaps John dozes, his old hand blanketing hers, for he returns to himself to find himself alone. His book is gone, burned or drowned or wandered to some other where, but a framed photograph rests on the seat of the chair beside his own. When he lifts it up to look at it, he sees a child smiling through the smutched glass at him. In the dim light, her features are none too clear, but he tilts the frame until he can view her face in the wedge of light that spills in from the hall.

The gap-toothed grin, the apprehensive eyes.

Her name was Miranda.

Miranda, with her love of stories and crayons, her understanding of endings. Miranda in the backseat of his car, begging him to member, claiming she did not like to get forgot. Miranda, his daughter, his sole and only child, the one for whom he'd once fashioned a lullaby from a dirge.

Miranda, John marvels, gazing into her dear face. He'd given her that name himself. Barb had wanted Jennifer or Amy or Nicole, but he'd held out for what he loved.

She'd had a gamin quality that he'd adored, when she was four and six and eight and even sixteen, a sly directness whose paradox enchanted him. When she was in grade school, he liked to pose her questions beyond her understanding—*What is the cause of thunder? What is honor? Is there any cause in nature that makes these hard hearts?* and he enjoyed the odd oracular quirkiness of her replies: *Birds' wings flapping. A risky pickle. The only cause is be.*

He used to coach her in memorizing lines, too. They'd started with *A Midsummer Night's Dream*—Lysander's gloomy disquisition on the course of true love, Bottom's revelation of his most rare dream, Puck's agile epilogue. He'd encouraged her with Cracker Jack. *Lord, what fools these mortals be!   Wonder on till truth make all things plain   A foolish heart, that I leave here behind   I know a bank where the wild thyme blows   If we shadows have offended*

She'd learned quickly, parroting the words she did not always understand, sometimes investing them with charming meanings of her own. *Wild thyme,* she'd claimed, was when it was okay to be loud and silly, and if, as her mother had recently explained, money did not grow on trees but came from banks instead, then it made sense for time to come from banks, too.

Miranda. He has always loved that name, coined by Shakespeare for the magician Prospero's daughter in the last full play he ever wrote. Miranda, from the Latin verb for wonder.

Though for Shakespeare, a wonder can be a calamity, a tragedy, or a disaster, too. *What is it you would see?* Horatio asks Prince Fortinbras in the final scene of *Hamlet* after the entire royal house of Denmark lies dead. *If aught of woe or wonder, cease your search.*

And now John recalls a calamitous Miranda, not Prospero's peerless daughter, but a girl more prone to disaster than to marvel. A strange changeling with purple hair and sullen shoulders, an angry wanton creature spitting curses at him. But despite all the ways she may have harmed him, despite the prickle of her demeanor and the folly of her garb, his old heart aches for her.

"I did her wrong," he says, looking past the smiling child to the scowling daughter beyond.

A woman slips up next to him in the darkling room, a gentle slip of a woman, sweet faced, brown skinned, her eyes alive in her dusky face.

"Mistah Wilson," she says, her voice like a warm breeze or a rich spice. "It's time for bed."

Sweetly, she guides him out of his chair and into the bathroom, sweetly helps him to undo his buttons and find his way into a pair of pajamas, sweetly helps to ease him between the sheets. Moved by her slender fingers and the softness of her voice, John accepts her ministrations almost gratefully, suffers her to set him aright.

"Good night," she says, bestowing one last smile, and then moving to close the curtains.

"Leave," John cries, "the, channel. I mean"—he waves an impatient hand in front of his face as if he were batting a cloud of gnats—"the . . . arras."

"Arras?" Puzzled, the woman turns towards him. "Perhaps you mean de curtain?"

"Curtain," he nods, accepting the word from her and then claiming it as his own. "Curtain."

Reaching for the cord that hangs from the rod, the woman pulls, and the curtains part again, gathering in pleats at either side to expose the opaque black glass as if revealing a stage.

"Spread thy close curtain, love-performing night," John mutters, staring beyond the dark window into a past where a host of ghostly memories is already being conjured, scents and tastes and glimpses that shift like wafting scarves.

"'Dat runaway's eyes may wink, and Romeo leap to dese arms untalk'd of and unseen.'"

The woman's words tug him back from the brink of some distant moment. "I beg . . . your pardon?" he says, turning from the window to stare at her.

"Dat is Mr. Shakespeare. We study his plays in school, in Trinidad. 'Lovers can see to do dere amorous rites by dere own beauties, or—'"

"'—if love be blind, it best agrees with night,'" John finishes the line with her, their voices blending as easily as if they'd rehearsed the words together.

"'Come, civil night,'" he continues.

"'Thou sober-suited matron all in black,
And learn me how to lose a winning match,
Play'd for a pair of stainless maidenhoods.'"

"So lovely," the woman murmurs when he finishes reciting, and then she waits quietly, allowing the words to ripen further. A moment later she adds, "I do not recall wat comes next, but later Juliet says:

"'Give me my Romeo, and, wen I shall die,
Take him and cut him out in little stars,
And he will make de face of heaven so fine
Dat all de world will be in love wit night.'

"I always have loved dat especially," she says, the love glowing on her face. "'All de world will be in love wit night,'" she repeats, her voice pure, her diction, despite the music of her accent, precise, "'and pay no worship to de garish sun.'"

"'When *I* shall die,'" John muses, "I."

"I must go now," the woman says, laying a gentle hand on John's skeletal shoulder. He feels her touch through the fabrics of his clothes, light as a golden leaf. "But I will see you again tomorrow. It is good to have a friend wit whom to recall Mr. Shakespeare."

Lying in his truckle bed, John watches as moonlight spills across the floor, so still, so calm, so silver, such a gift. When he lets his eyes sink shut at last, it seems the room is filled with spirits, as if everyone he ever lost is somehow with him still, so many gentle ghosts and tender phantoms—even Happy Dog, tangled in the covers somewhere.

A faint light appears in the dark sky, a pale rainbow glow growing so gradually that at first John thinks it must simply be his fancy. But as he watches, the merest curve of white begins to edge above the wall. The moon, John thinks—or one of them—a fat, round moon, rising like a bulbous slow balloon.

A moon like a blessing, he marvels as he watches, a cool forgiving moon, casting its soothing light on everything. *gracious moon   watery wandering   pale-faced moon* Its shine eases John's eyes, turns the tide of his vexed mind. *Good Lord, how bright and goodly shines the moon!*

Still it continues its imperturbable ascent, gaining in girth as it emerges from behind the wall, drenching bushes, leaves, and grasses with its silvern glow. As John gazes, it reaches its widest diameter, and then it rises further, a portly, portentous moon, so near and large John thinks he's ne'er seen the like, a benign giant of a moon, its serene and sorrowing face so close he might reach out and caress its shimmery coolth with his old dry palm. *Moon*, he thinks, his head ahum with sounds and sights and splintered facts, the same changeable orb the Elizabethans believed to be the boundary between the tainted earthly world and the perfect heavens above.

He'd made a study of the moon once, back in graduate school. He'd written a paper on the moon in one of Shakespeare's plays, a comedy whose name tingles on John's tongue's tip like the taste of moonlight, although frown as he might, he cannot will that name into his mind.

But he can recall those hours at his desk, his furious midnight typing, cups dregged with coffee, open books circled round him like magicians' tomes, balled sheets of onion skin overflowing the wastebasket and littering the floor, the moon outside his window ignored as he balances the solitary joy of insight and discovery with the finicky work of fitting footnotes at the bottom of each page. How happy he'd been, conversing—or cavorting—with that luminous play. Had he ever truly known his own luck? he wonders now. Had he ever lived inside his life as fully as his life—and he—deserved?

The moon perches atop the wall like Humpty Dumpty before his great fall while John strains to name that numinous play he'd once mined for the moon, the play of lunatics, lovers, poets, and fairies, as illuminated by moonshine as the night that blooms right now beyond his chamber window. *Thou hast by moonlight at her window sung   I do wander every where, Swifter than the moon's sphere   ill-met by moonlight, proud Titania   Moonshine and Lion are left to bury the dead*

"'Now the hungry lion roars,'" John chants in a rumbling whisper, "'And the wolf behowls the moon.'" In his lonely throat, the words rouse a feeling sharp as a kind of thirst. When he continues, it's as if another voice has suddenly joined his own, a child's voice, piping across the years, adding its ghostly eager treble to his rumble. "'Whilst the screech-owl, screeching loud,

>"'Puts the wretch that lies in woe
>In remembrance of a shroud.'"

Now the moon floats free of the wall to hover in the darkness like a magician's trick, and the play's name pops into existence like a gold coin or a rabbit or an endless silk scarf—*Dream*, he thinks, gazing out the window in silvery contentment, *A Midsummer Night's*

dream

When he finally manages to scale the ivied wall and heave himself over to land on the other side, he is scraped and aching in nearly a dozen places, his palms raw, his elbows stinging, his knees wet with blood or dew, his foolish mask askew. Panting, he lies on his belly in the damp grass. His heart pounds powerfully and his lungs feel huge, his body suddenly so alive that all his hurts are merest trifles, his torn clothes only another testament to the size of his life, the quality of his love.

He tears off the mask, hurls it away into the darkness. Rolling over onto his back, he lets the cool air kiss his cheeks as he looks up into the night where a moon hangs ripening. He sees the dark shape of the wall he has just scaled, sees the looming palazzo with its empty balcony, sees the trees that rise around him, their tops all tipped with silver, and above the trees, the blessed moon herself, while he lies in the damp rough grass, inhaling the scent of crushed weeds and jasmine and night-ripening fruit. All around him crickets sing, their song swelling and reeling, inhaling and exhaling like another kind of breathing, an endless, glorious spiraling of sound.

Lying hidden in that forbidden orchard, he has never been so happy. Everything he's ever known or done is merely a prelude to this moment, his whole life suddenly imbued with meaning simply because it has led him there, each stale day redeemed by his presence in this dangerous, life-engendering place. And come what sorrow can, he hardly cares, because in this moment he is entire. And alive.

Suddenly, a door opens above him, releasing a stream of light into the night, and now a woman drifts out on that golden river to lean against the stone railing of the balcony. He sees her round, slim arms, sees the shine of her eyes, the sheen of her dark hair. When she speaks, he hears her ask the whole wide night what's in a name

ANOTHER DAY. OR PERHAPS the same one, in this welked and wayward time.

Or maybe a day that he has lived before, and is now returning to once more, since time has of late developed the cunning trick of curving back on itself, curling under or doubling over so that he can reinhabit certain moments as if he had never left them, while the rest of his life remains as yet unclaimed.

Or then again, perhaps this is the sum and total of his existence— this aching body slumped in this worn chair. Maybe this windowed gaol is all the world, and the scenes and images that drift through his mind are not memories gone ragged but only his imagination, roaming places and meeting people that have never been. Perhaps he has but slumbered here while these visions did appear. Or maybe he has already died, and this is the sleep that rounds his little life.

Which critic was it who claimed that tragedy derives both its sorrow and its horror from the fact that time moves in one direction only, so that nothing can ever be foreknown and everything that happens happens only once, so what's done can never be undone? For years John found that a fine insight, useful in his teaching, and sometimes even in his own work. But lately it seems he's learned the knack of sidestepping time—or perhaps time has learned to sidestep him—for it seems that more and more, events come and go without reference to chronology, moments dropping in or moving on like the odd cast of characters who wander through his bedchamber door.

For instance, the last time he looked out this picture window, he would have sworn the welkin was a vibrant blue, the tree beside the casement all leaved in gold. But now, a mere trice later, the sky is sodden gray, the branches barren sticks, the lawn a sullen, wintery green.

He has been thinking about *The Winter's Tale*—or trying to— thinking about *The Winter's Tale* and the rest of the romances, though his thoughts drift like fish in a glass fishbowl, meandering in lazy circles, hardly pausing when they reach some invisible wall before they turn to swim back another way, occasionally catching the light as they shift and twist so that they shimmer with a momentary loveliness before they float on past, slipping like minnows beyond his grasp.

He has been thinking about redemption and deception—or trying to—since even now, alone in this strange chamber, there are so many interruptions to his work. Rain splattering the window. Blowing leaves and flocks of wind-whipped birds. A drifting harridan. A pabbling man. Fresh towels. Another dram of med'cine to be quaffed.

Still he soldiers on. Still slogs through bog and quagmire, still strives to understand. Understanding matters. That's what he tells his children . . . or his pupils . . . perhaps his progeny . . . or prodigy . . . or his pups. He who dies with the most understanding wins.

But perhaps even that truth has drifted away, since in the end, in *Pericles* and *Cymbeline*, in *The Winter's Tale*, and *The Tempest*, and perhaps even in *King Lear*, forgiveness and reconciliation seem to matter even more. *Forget and forgive,* say chastened Lear and compassionate Cleomenes. Others say it, too.

Forget.

And then forgive.

I like your silence, it the more shows off Your wonder. That's what grave and good Paulina says in the last scene of *The Winter's Tale* when she draws the curtain to reveal the statue Hermione has been for sixteen dreary years. And maybe, John muses, as the branches whip the sky and rain slaps its drops against the glass, Hermione speaks so little after she is stone no more not because she has been silenced by her husband's rage but because she's learned the value of wonder.

The next time John sees Will, he means to ask him that.

A woman comes to see him sometimes—and sometimes even now. A lined, warm woman in bright sweaters and worn jeans that invite him even now to ponder her dear bum. *Bum*, for the sum of the buns, and *buns* for both sweet cheeks, such fun bundles of language, such satisfying puns. There is no *fun* in Shakespeare, though. It's not a word he had, nor a word he ever had need of coining. For him, *joy*, *delight*, and *happiness* sufficed.

John is happy to be visited by that kind and handsome woman, delighted to have her company in these strange quarters, though she often strikes him as an epiphany come too late. He has never loved a woman so wholly before, but he wishes he could have loved her better, loved her sooner, loved her even more and longer than the small forever he's been given with her.

She seems fond of him, too, seems actually quite to dote. For that reason alone he knows he must be careful, for he wants never to break another heart.

"You," he tells her when she comes, "you are, my. You."

Then he pats her hand. Wordlessly.

Wordlessly, he studies her face, searches her eyes for meanings, for understandings. He'd forgotten—or had he ever known?—how naked a face could be, how open and expressive, how exposed. He'd never known—or had he forgotten?—how utterly one human could love another. Love beyond love.

Understanding may come hereafter.

Gusts of feeling or even thought still sometimes come, arriving like a wind rippling the calm surface of a stream.

Gently down the stream—he sang that once. With a child, a girl of five or six. *Row, row, row.* He remembers nodding and tapping her shoulder, cuing her when to begin, remembers smiling his encouragement for her to keep singing, to stick to her own words, keep to her own tune. *Life is but a dream.* He remembers her gleeful laughter when they reached the end.

A round, he'd said. *Let's sing a round.*

Or was he the child?

Remember, he thinks. He should—

But it seems his too, too solid mind is melting, thawing, resolving itself into a dew.

Adieu.

Adieu, adieu, remember me. The ghost says that, in *Hamlet.* And whether it is an honest ghost or not, each reader must discover for himself.

Reade him.

A woman arrives.

On this wet and wind-lashed day when trees are growing in the hallways and the ancientry croon about hark the herald angels and laughing all the way. The outside weather clings to her. Her chilled skin when she bends to kiss his pate, the rain sheen in her rumpled locks. Her hair is a plain chestnut color, a fact that pleases him inordinately, and for no good reason. Her countenance pleases him, too. Looking at her unremarkable young face, he feels a surge of gladness. He remembers those eyes, although he cannot say why. He remembers remembering them.

Déjà vu again.

That's an old joke. He smiles at it now, recalling someone making it and the others laughing, a band of young men in a dusky tavern. He tastes the hoppy sizzle of ale, cold and golden in his mouth, swipes the foam off his lip with a rugged wrist.

At the sight of his smile, the woman smiles, too. "Hi, Dad," she says. "I'm back again. Me and my foolish heart," she adds as if making a joke she expects him to understand. Deliberate as a judge, he watches as she flops into the chair beside his own, watches as she greets the gray world beyond the glass, the rain now dashing slant against the pane.

Waits until she parts the air between them to take his hand.

Now their linked fingers lie in his lap like a small warm animal, a pet that might need feeding.

"Give me your hands, if we be friends," he says, marveling at the finger pile, some straight-knuckled, others skewed and knobbled, the way they all accommodate each other, even so.

"'And Robin shall restore amends,'" the woman replies, her voice bright. "That's Puck, from *A Midsummer Night's Dream*. You taught me that, Dad, back when I was a girl. 'If we shadows have offended, think but this, and all is ended.'"

"*Mended*," he says, giving the mingled fingers in his lap a little shake. "'All is . . . *mended*.' Remember. There is no, *end*."

"Mended," she echoes, dutifully. "'All is mended.'"

That you have but slumb'red here While these visions did appear. He is so glad to see her. He has been waiting his whole life, it seems, for her to come. He would tell her that, if only he could recall her name. He can feel it shimmering on the tip of his mental tongue. And yet, like Hamlet's ghost, it vanishes when he calls. And whatever history he had with her now seems so distant, like the review of a play he has never actually seen, like the plot to *Two Noble Kinsmen* or *King John*, like poor young William Page's Latin declensions in *The Merry Wives of Windsor*: *Forsooth, I have forgot.*

"I thought we could give it one last try." The smile that trembles on her face is a lovely, delicate thing, a butterfly on this deep winter day.

"One," he tries, testing the word, curious to see where it might take him. A thought flits across his face. "There's something." He frowns. "I was going to . . . tell, something . . . to say."

"Yeah?"

"Something . . ." he gropes, "it was . . . matterful." But though he frowns and strains, in the end he has to sigh, "It's gone."

"It's okay, Dad." Her hand hugs his. "It doesn't matter. Or if it does—it'll come back later."

"When I'm . . . gone," he answers, though he sounds more wry than sorry. And yet a thought descends, pat as another deus ex machina. "Still . . . in coffee?"

"I am," she answers ebulliently. "But not for long. I have great news, Dad. I'm going to college, after all. I won that scholarship, the one I told you I'd never have a chance to get. For a game concept I came up with. It's called *Green World*."

"Green?" he asks the barren tree and blowing rain.

"*Green World*. You gave me the idea, Dad. How green worlds make people change, how confusion leads to transformation, and we have to leave our known safe lives before we can become anything really new. I worked those ideas into a concept for a game about how art and nature mirror and question each other, how humans are the interface between them. It's about finding a way to come to terms with chaos, and holding on to what matters, even as we let it go."

Her words are enigmatical, but her happiness is palpable, and he delights in it.

"I watched loads of plays online," she prattles. "I read a bunch, too. Sally sent me your teaching copies, with all your notes. She said I could keep them. Maybe I'll show them to my kids someday." Her talk is like a brook, a sparkling babble he does not need to understand. He trusts there is some wisdom in it, nonetheless.

"I like Sally," she says. "We've talked some on the phone. I'm headed off to ArtTech in a few days, but I'll be back for spring break, and we're planning on getting together then. Mink—that's my fiancé—he wants to learn about bees."

Afterwards, she sits in her car, sobbing a painful happiness while rain rattles the metal roof and tears drip off her chin to spot her coat.

"You sure about this, Ran?" Mink had asked before she left, his concern a treasure she trusts will never tarnish.

"Not sure at all," she'd answered tersely. Sighing carefully as if to avoid jostling her resolve, she'd added, "I only know I'm headed off to college in a few weeks, and there's a good chance I'll never see my dad again."

"But haven't you already said good-bye to him, like about a million times?"

"Maybe that's why I think it'll probably be okay whatever happens now." When he'd looked skeptical, she'd said, "Think about it like this: visiting him again is nothing compared to what I'll be doing next. Living away from you for the next four years, taking all those programming classes, a girl trying to break into—and then out of—the gamers' world. If I can do all that, I'm sure I can make one last visitation to dear old Dad.

"Besides," she went on with a sly smile, "I do kind of want to tell him to his face that it's thanks to him—and his Will—that I'm going to ArtTech after all."

It was on the drive home after her last visit that the idea came to her. Distraught at having lost her father and her last chance at ArtTech in a single hour, she'd spent the first twenty miles sobbing and swearing. As the road wound through the lush vineyards where the grape harvest had just begun, she'd held loud conversations with the father in her head, yelling and pleading, accusing, cursing, and beseeching.

By the time she'd joined the freeway, she'd mourned and ranted her way through the fiercest of her outrage and her grief. Rubbing away her tears, she'd driven in silence, too sorry to even turn the radio on, while her thoughts kept tugging helplessly back to her visit, the pity and the absurdity of it, and even the odd moments of interest: Cressida, dead white man's game, green worlds.

Green worlds—she'd brooded, gazing at the truck heaped with grapes that she was following—it sounded like the name for a computer game. And merely to distract herself and keep her losses at bay, she'd begun to imagine what a game called *Green World* might contain.

She'd begun working on it because it was her absolute final chance, but once she got inside it, she forgot about her chances, thought only of the promise of the game. Abandoning any hope of winning, she'd worked doggedly, steadily, but with a hot ferocious passion—sketching out ideas till dawn more nights than not, working until the work itself came to sustain her, until her love for what she was creating mattered more than any other prize.

She plundered Shakespeare's comedies and his romances, streaming videos and watching DVDs. She'd tried to read the plays and to read about them, combing the Internet and venturing into the UCSC library to learn more. There'd been much she hadn't understood and much more she hadn't understood well. But there'd been marvels, too, things that moved her or made her think—gems and joys and heart-stopping jabs.

Some of her searches led to her father's work, his articles, his books, his ideas referenced in other people's writing. Learning his thoughts by reading them, she felt again the ache of all she'd missed.

But she found him, too, in some strange way. She discovered in his writing his own passion and his care. Reading him, she'd seen he'd been much more than just her father, failed or not. And the more she read of him, the more she'd begun to believe he had tried harder as a father—and suffered more—than she had ever given him credit for.

A blast of wind buffets her car, sends water bucketing across the windshield. With a final sob, she digs the tears from her eyes and wipes her face.

Bequeath to death your numbness   *be stone no more.* The words arise in her mind like a distant lovely scent or a half-remembered tune. She's not sure where they come from, which character or what play, and yet they seem to fit so well all that she is feeling.

An old man sits. In the great churn of now.

An old man sits as the sun widens and the green returns.

No John at all, but just a picture window through which the world blows, a wind hole. Nothing left but sensations raining softly down around him, petaling, leafing, lighting and shadowing. A lifetime of sensations, drenching him. On this strange spring day that seems to have sprung from nowhere.

Green light flutters against pale green walls. Outside, the world ticks on, indifferent to any gaze. The bricks stand tall. The ivy curtain hangs. Daffodils and tulips sway in their bright chorus line, and sparrows bound across the greensward like kernels of popping corn. White clouds wander overhead, towered citadels, whales and dragonish vapors that roam the sky like dreams. Or memories.

Sometimes a memory envelops him, even now. Diving into a green cool river. Watching his mother flour the cutting board. Pushing a squealing child on a swing. Most of those memories are shadowed things, shreds and whispers that elude him even as he tries to reach for them. But occasionally they still arrive precise as stories—memories polished by decades of remembering, remembrances so keen he lives them still.

There was a garden. Long before his mother's face grew gray. Back when every now was new. A garden swooning with lilacs, shining with daffodils. And he was in that garden, he is in it still—not remembering, not staring through stiff glass or squinying back through time—but standing in its lemonade light, inhaling its dizzy scents, wrapped in its warm hum. Little Johnny, wrapped and rapt.

Everything is busy, lazy, buzzy. He sees his own white knees, the mocha dirt, sees the rainbows the sun makes when he squints his eyes half shut.

He sees his mother, in her polka-dot dress. She comes humming, sweeps him up. "A round," she says, smiling into his eyes, nodding, her face encouraging him while her voice sings, *Row, row, row your boat*— "Now you begin," she interrupts her singing to say.

"Row, row, row," he tries, his voice high and happy, but then he hears her words and gets confused. Fumbling, he loses track, sings her part instead *gently down   merrily   merrily   life   stream   but a   dream*

He stops, hot and flustered. But then she laughs and then he laughs, a round of laughter that erases his shame. The bee hum spins honey, the sound a kind of stream, another dream. *merrily   merrily   merrily* And he is once again so happy inside that buzzing singing laughing shining garden that there is no part of him left to think it. He is happy. Because. He is.

our little life Is rounded with a sleep. That's what the sage and sometime mage Prospero has to say.   *We are such stuff As dreams are made on   be cheerful, sir. Our revels now are ended.   Be not disturb'd with my infirmity.*

A woman comes, a young woman with a bright countenance and tousled hair. A woman he loves dearly, although he knows not why. Together they walk out of his cell into springtime, air warm as bathwater, world alive with daffodils that come before the swallow dares. And grass, newly grown and mown. The smell of green. Bees bumble by, their lulling hum. Birds flit and twitter. He shuffles down the sidewalk, her hand warm on his arm. A gift. A miracle. The present. They move slowly, one small step and then another. When he pauses, she waits. "It's good to be . . . home," he says, a full sentence, comprehensible. She saves it as a treasure.

Together they shuffle forward until they reach a pair of chairs.

"Would you like to sit?" she asks. Her voice is soft, gentle, and low. *An excellent thing*, he thinks, giving a slow, judicious nod. She helps to maneuver him toward his seat, steadies his upper arm as he lets himself thud down. "There you go," she says.

In response he farts, loud and long.

"Well roared, Lion," she gleeks. He nods again, serene.

They sit together, waiting.

A crow lands on the fresh grass, cocks its glossy head to consider them with a brazen eye.

"Up . . . start," he mutters. The rumble of his voice startles the bird, and it hops back into the air, catches itself on black wings, lumbers skyward.

They giggle together, father and daughter. The air heals.

After a while the waiting ceases, and they simply sit, the same breeze ruffling his grand white hair and her rumpled brown. Time dissolves.

He feels the breeze, its fingerless caress, watches the green lawn where an entire universe thrives—insects, microbes, bacteria, worms— all busy and oblivious, the mindless mind of the world.

He knows a sweep of gratitude, soft as another voice, and so wide and deep he believes he might drown in it. But he feels fearless, too, ready to be swept away on that unceasing current. Sitting with this woman who was—who is—so precious, though he cannot form the thought of why.

"So strange," he murmurs.

"What?" she asks almost languidly.

"That we . . ." He lifts his arm in a generous wide gesture, a blithe circle. "Are. What's so . . ." He lets his hand settle softly back in his lap like a petal dropping from a rose. "Is.

"I'll be leaving soon," he announces suddenly, more talkative than he's been in weeks.

"Leaving?" she echoes, leaning in. "Oh, Dad—"

He frowns a fatherly stern warning. "I must, not. Say no."

"Okay," she answers at last, taking his hand in hers. "All right."

"Each . . . breeze," he says, watching the ripple of the bright, unfurling leaves, "will be me, missing. You."

Smiling ruefully, she plays along, "And who says that, Dad? What character? Which play?"

"Play?" he echoes, perplexed. He shakes his head, momentarily nearly disturbed. "No . . . play." Gazing into her eyes at the green world reflected there, he answers, "Only, I."

THE END

Acknowledgments

Great thanks to my stalwart early readers: Cal Barksdale, Marc Bojanowski, Hannah Fisher, Ray Holley, Sharon O'Dair, Ken Rodgers, Neal Swain, Sean Swift, Patti Trimble—and especially Susan M. Gaines, Gayle Greene, and Elizabeth Wales.

And to my extended family's four generations of Shakespeare aficionados: Leonard and Virginia Hegland; Douglas Fisher; Hannah Fisher and Alex Voorhies; Tessa and Maggie Padilla Fisher; Garth Fisher; Heather Fisher and Russell, Ella, Clara, Lily and Celeste Shapiro; Caleb Thompson; Robert Thompson and Melanie Thornton; Aaron Rosewater; Adele Levin; and Renee, Kurt, Anya, and Georgia Mammen.